Insight in Medical Microbiology & Parasitology

MUHAMED T OSMAN

AYE AYE MON

MOHD WISMAN ABDUL HAMID

GHADA I. AL-DUBONI

DEDICATION

This book is dedicated to the students who have been a source of continuous stimulation and to our well-wishers in academic arena.

Osman, Aye, Wisman, and Ghada

CONTENTS

PREFACE

With the advent of rapid and amazing advances and recent break throughs in various fields of medicine in this millennium, including molecular aspects, genetics, epigenomics, and immunology the literature is inundated with considerable number of books, journals and raving reviews. But regrettably it is rather distressing to note the comparative deficiency of books and guides on evaluation of medical undergraduates paripassu with the magnitude of ever mounting literature on colossal breath taking advances enhancing comprehension of various disciplines of medicine. The relatively alarming dearth of guide books such as this the most useful instruments of evaluation dimensions of embedded knowledge in undergraduate medical students, has prompted publication of this book. This book contains 375 questions dealing with all important topics of Medical Microbiology including Bacteriology, Virology, Mycology and Clinical Microbiology in addition to Medical Parasitology.

This will surely serve as an excellent tool for self- appraisal as well as a stimulus for gauging one's abilities to analyze, rationalize and synthesize the knowledge. In fact it can even be effectively utilized for group discussions among students which verily would foster their maturity and academic advancement. If this is found useful it would confirm our aspirations as not only teachers and trainers but testers as well. We wish all the readers a salubrious journey through this book which is a compulsory companion to all students. We wish to acknowledge with gratitude all those colleagues who participated in the preparation of this one way or other and particularly students who were the driving force.

1 BACTERIOLOGY

1.1 Questions without answers: (True/False Questions) :

1. **Robert Koch:**

    A. discovered that injected pure cultures of anthrax bacilli into mice and caused anthrax.
    B. investigated the aetiology of tuberculosis.
    C. developed the first antibiotic that selectively killed the pathogen.
    D. formulated Koch's postulates.
    E. introduced antiseptic surgery.

2. **Discoveries of Louis Pasteur included:**

A. Microorganisms are the causes of infectious disease.
B. Technique of pasteurization.
C. Vaccine against anthrax.
D. Penicillin.
E. Microscope.

3. Therapeutics include:

A. Drugs.
B. Surgery.
C. radiation therapy.
D. Tattooing.
E. Psychiatry.

4. Plasmids:

A. are small circular extra-chromosomal DNA.
B. sizes vary from 1 to 1,000 kilobase pairs.
C. found in eukaryotes.
D. found in prokaryotes.
E. not associated with mechanism of gene transfer.

5. Autoclave can be used in sterilization of:

A. laboratory glassware.
B. surgical instruments.
C. Paraffin.
D. Powders.
E. rubber gloves.

6.   Bacteria

A.   are single- cell eukaryotes.

B.   have true nucleus.

C.   have rigid cell wall containing peptidoglycan.

D.   are classified according to shape, gram staining reaction, oxygen requirement.

E.   can grow on inanimate culture medium.

7.   The characteristics of bacteria include:

A.   being haploid.

B.   division by binary fission.

C.   having no nuclear membrane.

D.   multicellular eukaryotes with no rigid cell wall.

E.   unicellular organisms with prokaryotic cell structures.

8.   Spore forming bacteria are

A.   *Clostridium difficile.*

B.   *Corynebacterium diptheriae.*

C.   *Bacillus anthracis.*

D.   *Clostridium tetani.*

E.   *Bacillus cereus.*

9   Regarding structure of bacteria, the following means::

A.   Spherical or oval = cocci.

B.   rod-shaped = vibrios.

C.   flexous, spiral = spirochaetes.

D.   comma-shaped = actinomycetes.

E.   helical & cylindrical = bacilli.

10   For cultivation of bacteria, the followings should be considered:

A.   choosing appropriate specimen to examine.
B.   specimen should avoid contamination from normal flora.
C.   prompt transportation of the specimen to the laboratory.
D.   essential information about antibiotic.
E.   none of the above.

11   The following statements are true for bacteria:

A.   They possess rigid cell wall.
B.   They are motile by means of pseudopodia.
C.   They cannot be grown on artificial media.
D.   They multiply by binary division.
E.   Almost all bacteria can form spore.

12   Bacteria that can grow either in the presence or absence of oxygen are called:

A.   facultative anaerobes.
B.   Microaerophiles.
C.   strict anaerobes.
D.   obligate aerobes.
E.   obligate anaerobes.

13   Sodium hypochlorite is

A.   used for viral environmental disinfection.

B.   used on smooth and hard surfaces of the floor.

C.   not a useful disinfectant for laboratory discard jars.

D.   caustic to the skin at high concentration.

E.   an effective disinfectant for *Mycobacterium tuberculosis.*

14   The virulence of the organisms is determined by

A.   presence of fimbriae.

B.   presence of metachromatic granules.

C.   production of toxin.

D.   presence of spores.

E.   production of aggressive enzymes.

15   Antibiotic resistance among bacteria

A.   occurs by altering the number and structure of porins.

B.   is attributed to plasmids.

C.   is estimated by staining techniques.

D.   is transmitted by virulent bacteriophages.

E.   occurs due to alteration of target sites on the bacteria.

16   The following are statements regarding events of bacterial morphology:

A.   The name spirillum refers to rod-like bacteria.

B.   The name coccus refers to spherical like bacteria.

C.   Bacteria form distinctive cell morphologies when grown on Petri plates.

D.   Bacteria form distinct colony morphologies when examined by light microscopy.

E.   Some bacteria produce elaborate structures bearing

reproductive spores (e.g. Myxococcus).

17 The following are statements regarding the primary structure of bacterial biological macromolecules:

A. The sequence in which the subunits are put together in the macromolecule is called the primary structure.
B. Primary structure determines many of the properties that the macromolecule will have.
C. Majority of amino acids of proteins are found in membranes.
D. Carbohydrates of polysaccharides are found in capsules, inclusions (storage) and cell walls.
E. tRNA is found in cytoplasm.

18 The following are statements regarding bacterial cell wall:

A. It provides structural integrity to the bacterial cell.
B. Peptidoglycan is responsible for the determination of cell shape.
C. Several antibiotics stop bacterial infections by interfering with cell wall synthesis.
D. For both Gram-positive and Gram-negative bacteria, particles of approximately 2 nm can pass through the peptidoglycan.
E. If the bacterial cell wall is entirely removed, it is called a spheroplast.

19 The following are statements regarding bacterial cell wall:

A. It is an essential structure for viability.
B. It is composed of many different components.
C. It is one of the most important sites for attack by antibiotics.

D.   It causes symptoms of disease in animals.

E.   It provides for immunological distinction and immunological variation among strains of bacteria.

20   **The bacterial cell structures are correctly matched with their functions:**

A.   Cell wall of Gram-positive bacteria : Prevents osmotic lysis of cell protoplast and confers rigidity and shape on cells.

B.   Common pilli or fimbriae : protection against phagotrophic engulfment.

C.   Plasma membrane   : energy generation and location of numerous enzyme systems.

D.   Ribosomes   : Sites of translation (protein synthesis)

E.   Plasmid   :   Extrachromosomal genetic material.

21   **The following major elements are correctly matched with general physiological functions :**

A.   Oxygen   : Constituent of cell material.

B.   Carbon   : Main constituent of cellular material.

C.   Nitrogen   : Constituent of amino acids, nucleic acids nucleotides, and coenzymes.

D.   Hydrogen   : Main constituent of organic compounds and cell water.

E.   Iron :   Main cellular inorganic cation and cofactor for certain enzymes.

22   **The following common vitamins required in the nutrition of certain bacteria are correctly matched with following functions**

A. Folic acid   :   required for synthesis of purine bases and methionine.
B. Biotin   : Biosynthetic reactions that require CO_2 fixation.
C. Nicotinic acid : Electron carrier in dehydrogenation reactions.
D. Vitamin K   : Electron transport processes.
E. Thiamine (B_1) : Transfer of methyl groups.

23   **The following methods used to measure bacterial growth are correctly matched with their applications**

A. Direct microscopic count : Enumeration of bacteria in milk or cellular vaccines.
B. Viable cell count (colony counts) : Enumeration of bacteria in milk, foods, soil, water, laboratory cultures, etc.
C. Turbidity measurement : Microbiological assays.
D. Measurement of dry weight or wet weight of cells or volume of cells after centrifugation : Measurement of total cell yield in cultures.
E. Measurement of total N or protein : Measurement of total cell yield from very dense cultures.

24   **The following are statements regarding methods used to measure bacterial growth:**

A. Direct microscopic count can distinguish living from nonliving cells.
B. Colony counts are very sensitive if plating conditions are optimal.
C. Turbidity measurement is slow and destructive.
D. Measurement of total N or protein is only practical application is in the research laboratory.
E. Measurement of Biochemical activity Requires a fixed

standard to relate chemical activity to cell mass and/or cell numbers.

25   The following method used to measure bacterial growth is correctly matched with its application:

A.   Direct microscopic count : Enumeration of bacteria.

B.   Viable cell count (colony counts) : Enumeration of bacteria

C.   Turbidity measurement : Estimations of large numbers of bacteria in clear liquid media and broths.

D.   Measurement of total N or protein : Measurement of total cell yield from very dense cultures.

E.   Measurement of dry weight or wet weight of cells or volume of cells after centrifugation : Measurement of total cell yield in cultures.

26   The following Medium is used in generation for some common bacteria under optimal conditions of growth :

A.   Glucose-salts *: Escherichia coli.*

B.   Sucrose-salts *: Bacillus megaterium.*

C.   Heart infusion broth *:   Staphylococcus aureus.*

D.   Milk *: Lactobacillus acidophilus .*

E.   Mannitol-salts-yeast extract *:   Treponema pallidum .*

27   The following are statements regarding bacterial mutants:

A.   Mutants in bacteria are mostly biochemical in nature.

B.   Auxotrophs are the most important mutants.

C.   Chemoauxotrophs are mutants that can't use some nutrient (usually a sugar) that prototrophs can use as food.

D. Drug resistance mutants are usually dominant.

E. Auxotrophs and chemoauxotrophs are usually recessive.

28 The following are statements regarding bacterial sexual processes:

A. Conjugation is a direct transfer of DNA from one bacterial cell to another.

B. Transduction is the use of a bacteriophage to transfer DNA between cells.

C. Transformation is a naked DNA is taken up from the environment by bacterial cells.

D. In transformation the E. coli cells are made "competent" to be transformed by treatment with calcium ions and heat shock.

E. The transduction is the closest analogue in bacteria to eukaryotic sex.

29 Significance of plasmids include

A. codes for resistance to several antibiotics like Gram-negative bacteria carry plasmids that give resistance to antibiotics such as penicillins..

B. codes for the production of toxins (such as Enterotoxins by *Escherichia coli*)

C. codes for resistance to heavy metals such as Hg.

D. plasmids carry virulence determinant genes. Eg, the plasmid Col V of *Escherichia coli* contains genes for iron sequestering compounds.

E. contains genes coding for enzymes that allow bacteria unique or unusual materials for carbon or energy sources.

30   The physiological mechanisms of antibiotic resistance include

    A.   activation of the antibiotic by enzymes produced by the bacteria.

    B.   alteration of target proteins such that the antibiotic doesn't bind or binds with decreased affinity.

    C.   alteration of the membrane which decreases the permeability of the antibiotic.

    D.   active efflux of the antibiotic.

    E.   development of alternate metabolic pathway to bypass the action of antibiotic.

31   The following examples of bacteria are correctly matched with a method of adhesion to host cell or tissue surfaces:

    A.   *Streptococcus pyogenes* :   Protein F.

    B.   *Streptococcus mutans*:   Cell-bound protein .

    C.   *Neisseria gonorrhoeae* :   Type IV pili (N-methylphenyl-alanine pili)

    D.   *Enterotoxigenic E. coli*   :   Type-I fimbriae.

    E.   Mycoplasma :   Membrane protein.

32   The following extracellular bacterial proteins invasins are correctly matched with types of bacteria:

    A.   Hyaluronidase : Streptococci .

    B.   Phospholipases *: Clostridium* species .

    C.   Coagulase *: Staphylococcus aureus* .

    D.   Lecithinases *: Clostridium perfringens* .

    E.   Neuraminidase *: Vibrio cholerae* .

33 **The following are statements regarding comparison between properties of bacterial endotoxins and classic exotoxin:**

A.   relationship to cell is part of outer membrane in endotoxin while it is extracellular in ebdotoxin.

B.   endotoxin is usually denatured by boiling while not in exotoxin.

C.   Both are antigenic.

D.   Both can converted to toxoids.

E.   endotoxins are less potent while exotoxins are relatively high potency.

34 **The following bacterial exotoxins are correctly with their biological effects:**

A.   Cholera toxin   :   Activates adenylate cyclase; increased level of intracellular cAMP promote secretion of fluid and electrolytes in intestinal epithelium leading to diarrhea.

B.   Diphtheria toxin : Inhibits protein synthesis resulting in death of the cells.

C.   *E. coli* heat-labile toxin LT : Blocks inhibition of adenylate cyclase; increased levels of cAMP affect hormone activity and reduce phagocytic activity.

D.   *Pseudomonas* Exotoxin A : Inhibits protein synthesis in susceptible cells, resulting in death of the cells.

E.   *Staphylococcus aureus* Exfoliatin B : Separation of the stratum granulosum of the epidermis, between the living layers and the superficial dead layers.

35 **The following pore-forming bacterial toxins are correctly matched with the diseased caused:**

A. perfringiolysin O from *Clostridium perfringens* : gas gangrene.
B. Hemolysin from *Escherichia coli* : diarrhoea .
C. alpha toxin from *Staphylococcus aureus* : abcesses.
D. streptolysin O from *Streptococcus pyogenes* : strep throat.
E. Leukocidin from Staphylococcus aureus : pyogenic infections.

36 The followings characteristics are generally present in a Gram-positive bacterium:

A. cytoplasmic lipid membrane.
B. teichoic acids in the cell wall.
C. capsule polysaccharides (only in some species)
D. flagellum(only in some species)
E. the transpeptidase creates a covalent bond directly between peptidoglycan molecules, with no intervening bridge.

37 The following are statements regarding Gram-positive bacteria:

A. They are able to retain the crystal violet stain because of their thick peptidoglycan.
B. Plasma membrane, PG layer and cell wall are three distinct structures.
C. They are amorphous and can change shape, since the outer plasma membrane consists of a dynamic lipid bilayer.
D. The S-layer is attached to directly to the outer membrane.
E. They are bounded by a single unit lipid membrane.

38 The following are statements regarding Gram-negative

bacteria:

A. In a Gram stain test, a counterstain (commonly safranin) is added after the crystal violet, coloring all gram-negative bacteria with a red or pink color.
B. They are less resistant than gram-positive bacteria against antibiotics.
C. The pathogenic capability of them is often associated with certain components of cell envelope, in particular, the lipopolysaccaride.
D. Gram-negative bacteria associated with nosocomial infections.
E. The proteobacteria are a major group of them.

39 The following characteristics are generally present in a Gram-negative bacteria:

A. Thick peptidoglycan layer.
B. Outer membrane containing lipopolysaccharide.
C. There is a space between the layers of peptidoglycan and the secondary cell membrane called the periplasmic space.
D. The S-layer is directly attached to the outer membrane, rather than the peptidoglycan.
E. No teichoic acids.

40

Gram-negative Bacteria vs Gram-positive Bacteria

	Gram-negative Bacteria	**Gram-positive Bacteria**
A.	Peptidoglycan layer is thin.	Peptidoglycan layer is thick.
B.	Outer membrane is absent.	Outer membrane is present.

C.	Lipid and lipoprotein content is high.	Lipid and lipoprotein content is low.
D.	Toxins produced is primarily endotoxins.	Toxins produced is primarily extotoxins.
E.	More resistance to antibiotics.	More susceptible to antibiotics.

41 **The following are statements regarding virulence factors of *S. aureus*:**

A. surface proteins promote colonization of host tissues.
B. invasins promote bacterial spread in tissues.
C. surface factors damage host tissues or provoke symptoms of disease.
D. biochemical properties enhance their survival in phagocytes.
E. membrane-damaging toxins lyse eucaryotic cell membranes.

42 **The following are statements regarding *Streptococcus pyogenes* (Group A streptococcus):**

A. It is a Gram-negative bacteria.
B. The metabolism of S. pyogenes is fermentative.
C. It requires enriched medium containing blood in order to grow.
D. Group A streptococci typically have a capsule composed of hyaluronic acid and exhibit beta (clear) hemolysis on blood agar.
E. M protein is a virulence factor of it.

43 **The following are statements regarding *Escherichia coli*:**

A. It is facultatively anaerobic Gram-negative rods.

B. It can grow in media with glucose and additional growth factors.
C. It is a consistent inhabitant of the human intestinal tract.
D. P fimbriae are used in adhesion.
E. Pathogenic strains of E. coli are responsible for neonatal meningitis.

44 The following are statements regarding diseases caused by *Streptococcus pyogenes:*

A. Suppurative condition occur in the throat.
B. Streptococcal pharyngitis is acquired by inhaling aerosols emitted by infected individuals.
C. Impetigo is the infection of the dermis.
D. Scarlet fever is caused by production of erythrogenic toxin by a few strains of the organism.
E. Toxic shock is caused by a few strains that produce a toxic shock-like toxin.

45 The following are statements regarding *Streptococcus* *pneumoniae***:**

A. It is a normal inhabitant of the human lower respiratory tract.
B. *Streptococcus pneumoniae* cells are Gram-positive, lancet-shaped cocci.
C. They are alpha hemolytic when cultured on blood agar.
D. They do not form spores.
E. It causes osteomyelitis.

46 The following are statements regarding Gram-negative aerobic rods and cocci:

A. This group consists of Gram-negative bacteria phenotypically related to members of the genus *Pseudomonas*.
B. Their metabolism is fermentative.
C. Many bacteria in this group are free-living in soil and water.
D. *Pseudomonas aeruginosa* is a leading cause of hospital-acquired infections.
E. *Bordetella pertussis* causes of Whooping cough.

47 The following are statements regarding Enteric bacteria:

A. They are Gram-positive rods with facultative anaerobic metabolism.
B. This group consists of *Escherichia coli* and its relatives.
C. They all ferment glucose to acid end products.
D. They are consistent members of the normal flora.
E. *Shigella dysenteriae* causes bacillary dysentery.

48 The following are statements regarding *Pyogenic Cocci*:

A. The Gram-positive cocci produce at least a third of all the bacterial infections of humans.
B. *Staphylococcus aureus* occur normally on the nasal membranes.
C. *S. epidermidis* is rarely a pathogen.
D. *S. pyogenes* is coomonly found as normal flora in the upper respiratory tract.
E. *Streptococcus pneumoniae* is the most frequent cause of otitis media.

49 The following are statements regarding Endospore-forming

bacteria:

A. They are Gram-positive and usually rod-shaped.
B. *Bacillus anthracis* causes food poisoning.
C. *Clostridium perfringens* causes anaerobic wound infections and gas gangrene.
D. *Clostridium difficile* causes pseudomembranous colitis.
E. *Listeria monocytogenes* does not form endospore.

50 The following are statements regarding vibrios:

A. They are capable of both respiratory and fermentative metabolism.
B. They are distinguished from enterics by being oxidase-positive and motile by means of polar flagella.
C. In liquid media vibrios are motile by polar flagella.
D. *V. parahaemolyticus* is noninvasive, affecting the small intestine through secretion of an enterotoxin.
E. Treatment of cholera involves the rapid intravenous replacement of the lost fluid and ions.

51 The following are statements regarding Salmonella:

A. It is a Gram-negative facultative rod-shaped bacterium.
B. It is the cause of acute gastroenteritis, resulting from bacterial invasion of the bloodstream .
C. All *Salmonella* serovars form a single DNA hybridization group.
D. *Salmonella* typhi produce flagella.
E. Salmonellosis in these cases is transmitted through fecal contamination of water or food.

52   Characteristics of Salmonella include:

A.   Gram-positive bacteria.
B.   Lactose negative.
C.   Methyl red test positive.
D.   Citrate positive (growth on Simmon's citrate agar)
E.   Urease negative.

53   The following are statements regarding *Pseudomonas aeruginosa*:

A.   It is a free-living bacterium.
B.   It is primarily a nosocomial pathogen.
C.   It causes urinary tract infections.
D.   In the laboratory, the simplest medium for growth of *Pseudomonas aeruginosa* consists of acetate as a source of carbon and ammonium sulfate as a source of nitrogen.
E.   It is highly sensitive to many antibiotics.

54   The following are statements regarding Shigellae:

A.   They are Gram-negative, motile, non-spore forming, rod-shaped bacteria.
B.   Eosin methylene blue (EMB) agar is used to determine the bacteria.
C.   The primary plating media shown here are, MacConkey agar, ENDO agar, Hektoen enteric (HE) agar and Salmonella-Shigella (SS) agar.
D.   *Shigella dysenteriae* type 1, causes deadly epidemics in many developing countries.
E.   Ampicillin, is commonly used in treatment.

55 The following are statements regarding Actinobacteria:

A. They are a group of Gram-positive bacteria.
B. They have high guanine and cytosine content in their DNA.
C. Most Actinobacteria of medical significance are in subclass Actinobacteridae, order Actinomycetales.
D. Some Actinobacteria form branching filaments.
E. All actinobacteria are aerobic.

56 The following are statements regarding Mycobacterium:

A. They are aerobic.
B. Mycobacteria do not contain endospores or capsules.
C. They are classified as an acid-fast Gram-positive bacterium.
D. All *Mycobacterium* species have a characteristic thin cell wall.
E. Some species are very easy to culture.

57 The following are statements regarding Mycobacterium:

A. *M. tuberculosis* is nonpigmented in the light and dark.
B. Mycobacteria are classical acid-fast organisms.
C. Stains used in evaluation of tissue specimens or microbiological specimens include Ziehl-Neelsen stain.
D. Mycobacteria appear phenotypically most closely related to members of *Nocardia*, *Rhodococcus* and *Corynebacterium*.
E. All Mycobacteria are found as free-living bacteria.

58 The following are statements regarding anaerobes:

A. They are all Gram-positive.

B. They are commensal organisms of the mouth, oropharynx.

C. Infections with anaerobes are frequently polymicrobial.

D. Often associated with foul or putrid odour.

E. They are usually sensitive to clindamycin.

59 The following are statements regarding anaerobes:

A. They require molecular oxygen as a terminal electron acceptor.

B. Anaerobes cannot grow in the presence of oxygen.

C. Their metabolism is a fermentative type.

D. Many members of the indigenous human flora are anaerobic bacteria.

E. Infections produced by anaerobic bacteria occur in few parts of the human body.

60 The following are statements regarding Spirochaetes:

A. They are chemoheterotrophic in nature.

B. They are distinguished from other bacterial phyla by the type of cell membrane.

C. Most spirochaetes are anaerobic.

D. *Borrelia burgdorferi* causes Lyme disease.

E. *Borrelia recurrentis*, causes relapsing fever .

61 The following are statements regarding Spirochaetes:

A. They are easily observed by light microscope.

B. Most of them appear as helical coils.

C. Their flagella lie between the outer membrane and the peptidoglycan layer,

D. Nonpathogenic treponemes can be found in the oral cavity.

E. Penicillin is used for treatment of all stages of syphilis.

62 The following are statements regarding Chlamydia:

A. Chlamydia infections are the most common leading cause of infectious blindness worldwide.

B. The *Chlamydia suis* species is a human pathogen.

C. It is found in the form of an elementary body and a reticulate body.

D. Commonly Chlamydia infections cause symptoms.

E. Chlamydia is detected by fluorescent monoclonal antibody test.

63 The following are statements regarding Mycoplasma:

A. They are affected by many common antibiotics such as penicillin.

B. They can survive without oxygen.

C. Most of them are pseudococcoidal.

D. They are most require sterols for the stability of their cytoplasmic membrane.

E. *M. pneumoniae* is a cause of atypical pneumonia.

64 The following are statements regarding *Mycoplasma*:

A. *Mycoplasma* species are often found in research laboratories as contaminants in cell culture..

B. They are easily detected by conventional microscope.

   C.   Mycoplasmas may induce cellular changes, including chromosome aberrations.

   D.   Enzyme immunoassays is used in their detection.

   E.   Majority of mycoplasma infections in humans are associated with skin eruptions.

65   **The following are statements regarding *Ureaplasma urealyticum*:**

   A.   It is a bacterium belonging to the family Mycoplasmataceae.

   B.   It is part of the normal genital flora of both men and women

   C.   It has been noted as one of the infectious causes of sterile pyuria.

   D.   Cholesterol is required for their growth.

   E.   Penicillin is the drug of choice.

66   **The following are statements regarding Rickettsias:**

   A.   They are Gram-negative.

   B.   They divide by binary fission and they metabolize host-derived glutamate.

   C.   They can grow outside of a host cell.

   D.   They occur in nature in the gut lining of arthropods .

   E.   *Rickettsia rickettsii* is the cause of epidemic typhus.

67   **The following are statements regarding virulence of Rickettsiae:**

   A.   Rickettsiae are inoculated into the dermis of the skin by a tick bite or through damaged skin from the feces of lice or fleas.

   B.   The bacteria spread through the bloodstream and infect the endothelium.

C.   The adhesins are presumed to be outer membrane proteins.

D.   Typhus group rickettsiae are released from host cells by lysis of the cells.

E.   Spotted fever group rickettsiae accumulate in large numbers and do lyse the host cells.

68   The following are statements regarding *Orientia tsutsugamushi*:

A.   It is the causative organism of scrub typhus.

B.   Trombiculid mites is the natural vector and reservoir.

C.   Its envelope is similar to that of Gram positive bacteria.

D.   It is an obligatory intracellular organism.

E.   It is sensitive to doxycycline.

69   The following are statements regarding Ehrlichia:

A.   They are transmitted by ticks.

B.   They are obligately intracellular pathogens.

C.   They infect and kill red blood cells.

D.   Onset of its symptoms began exactly 14 days after bite occurred.

E.   Penicillin is the drug of choice.

70   The following are statements regarding *Bartonella*:

A.   *Bartonella* species are considered as opportunistic pathogens.

B.   Mammals are the reservoir hosts.

C.   Homeless IV drug users are at high risk for *Bartonella* infections.

D.   *Bartonella henselae* is the organism responsible for cat scratch disease.

E. *B. henselae* is generally susceptible to penicillin.

71 The following are statements regarding *Coxiella burnetii*:

A. It is the causative agent of Q fever.
B. It is susceptible to environmental stresses like uv light.
C. Inhalation of one organism will yield disease in 50% of the population.
D. Disease occurs as one stage of respiratory symptoms.
E. A combination of erythromycin and rifampin is highly effective in treatment.

72 *Staphylococci*

A. are catalase test negative.
B. are resistant to bacitracin.
C. are soil microbial flora.
D. do not grow in Mannitol salt agar.
E. grow in a 6.5% NaCl solution.

73 Spore forming bacteria include

A. *Haemophilus influenza.*
B. *Bacillus cereus.*
C. *Clostridiumdifficile.*
D. *Corynebacterium diphtheriae.*
E. *Rickettsia prowazekii.*

74 **The pathogenic conditions caused by *Klebsiella pneumoniae* include**

    A.   pyogenic skin infections.
    B.   pneumonia .
    C.   scarlet fever.
    D.   urinary tract infection.
    E.   wound infections.

75 *Clostridium difficile*

    A.   causes nosocomial diarrhoea.
    B.   infection is treated by amphotericin B.
    C.   is a gram negative bacilli.
    D.   is acquired by persons receiving clindamycin in the hospital.
    E.   is not a primary pathogen for pseudomembranous colitis.

76 *Mycobacterium tuberculosis*

    A.   causes leprosy in immunocompetent persons.
    B.   is an acid fast bacillus.
    C.   is commonly found in patient with HIV infection.
    D.   is transmitted by inhalation.
    E.   is treated by single drug therapy.

77 *Mycobacterium leprae*

    A.   was described by Hansen.
    B.   can be isolated in artificial culture media.
    C.   is seen as acid fast bacilli arranged in cigar bundle shape.
    D.   naturally infects armadillos.

E.   causes Lyme disease.

78   *Bacillus anthracis*

A.   is a spore-bearing bacilli.
B.   causes food poisoning.
C.   can be used as a potential biological weapon.
D.   infection occurs mainly in humans.
E.   is a strict anaerobe.

79   *Pseudomonas aeruginosa*

A.   is one of the nosocomial pathogens.
B.   produces blue colored pigments.
C.   can cause wound infection.
D.   is a Gram-positive spore forming bacillus.
E.   can be treated with tetracycline.

80   *Haemophilus influenzae*

A.   is a small gram-negative coccobacillus.
B.   can grow on ordinary culture media.
C.   is responsible for meningitis.
D.   is diagnosed by doing capsule swelling reaction test.
E.   is prevented by the vaccine.

81   The characteristic features of *Mycoplasma pneumoniae* include

A.   obligate intracellular organism.

B.   can cause atypical pneumonia.
C.   transmitted by sexual route.
D.   presence of rigid cell wall.
E.   completely sensitive to penicillin.

82   The virulence factors of *Streptococcus pyogenes* include

A.   lipotechoic acid which facilitates binding to respiratory epithelium.
B.   M-protein which is an adherence protein.
C.   presence of capsule which protects against phagocytosis.
D.   presence of flagella which assist in escaping host defense mechanisms.
E.   production of hyaluronidase which causes spreading cellulitis.

83   The following are statements regarding Lab diagnosis of bacterial infections:

A.   *Bacillus anthracis* appear on blood agar as large, grayish, nonhemolytic colonies with irregular borders.
B.   Brucella species are diagnosed by culture.
C.   *Chlamydia trachomatis* is diagnosed by cellular cytoplasmic inclusions by immunofluorescence technique.
D.   *Clostridium botulinum* is diagnosed by culture in standard aerobic culture.
E.   *Escherichia coli* (generally) Cultured on MacConkey agar and study carbohydrate fermentation patterns.

84   The following laboratory diagnostic methods are correctly matched with types of bacteria:

A. Culture on Tinsdale agar, followed by immunologic precipitin reaction : *Corynebacterium diphtheria.*

B. Culture in 6.5% NaCl : *Enterococcus faecalis.*

C. Culture on MacConkey agar : *Haemophilus influenza.*

D. Urease-positivity : *Helicobacter pylori.*

E. Serology for antibodies against O antigen : *Salmonella typhi.*

85 The following are statements regarding microbes that produce natural antibiotics:

A. *Cephalosporium* molds produce the base molecule for development of semisynthetic beta-lactam antibiotics.

B. *Streptomyces* species produce tetracyclines.

C. *Bacillus* species produce polypeptide antibiotics.

D. The maintenance of a substantial component of the bacterial genome devoted solely to the synthesis of an antibiotic.

E. Most of the microorganisms that produce antibiotics are sensitive to the action of their own antibiotic.

86 The following are statements regarding characteristics of antibiotics:

A. Spectrum of action is the range of bacteria or other microorganisms that is affected by a certain antibiotic.

B. Broad spectrum antibiotics are effective against procaryotes that kill or inhibit a wide range of Gram-positive and Gram-negative bacteria.

C. Narrow spectrum antibiotics are effective mainly against Gram-positive or Gram-negative bacteria.

D. Limited spectrum antibiotics are effective against a single organism or disease.

E.   A clinically-useful antibiotic should have a wide spectrum of activity with the ability to destroy or inhibit many pathogenic organisms.

87   A clinically-useful antibiotic should have as many of these characteristics as possible:

A.   It should be without undesirable side effects.
B.   It should be nonallergenic to the host.
C.   It should not eliminate the normal flora of the host.
D.   It should be chemically-stable (have a long shelf-life).
E.   Microbial resistance is common and likely to develop.

88   The following classes of antibiotics are correctly matched with their spectrum (effective against) :

A.   Beta-lactams (penicillins and cephalosporins) : Gram-positive bacteria.
B.   Semisynthetic beta-lactams : Gram-positive and Gram-negative bacteria.
C.   Clavulanic Acid : Gram-positive bacteria.
D.   Aminoglycosides   : Gram-positive and Gram-negative bacteria.
E.   Lincomycins : Gram-positive and Gram-negative bacteria esp. anaerobic *Bacteroides.*

89   The most important targets in bacteria by antibiotic :

A.   Bacterial cell wall synthesis.
B.   Interfere with protein synthesis.
C.   Interference with nucleic acid synthesis.

D. Inhibition of an essential metabolic pathway that exists in the bacterium .

E. Membrane inhibition or disruption works too well.

90 The following are statements regarding MRSA (methicillin/oxacillin-resistant Staphylococcus aureus):

A. It has evolved resistance not only to beta-lactam antibiotics, but to several classes of antibiotics.

B. Some MRSA are resistant to all but one or two antibiotics, notably vancomycin-resistant.

C. Hospital-Associated MRSA (HA-MRSA) occurs less frequently among patients who undergo invasive medical procedures.

D. The main mode of HA-MRSA transmission to other patients is through human hands.

E. Minority of Community-Associated MRSA (CA-MRSA) infections are localized to skin and soft tissue.

91 The following antibiotic is correctly matched with method of resistance:

A. Sulfonamides : metabolic bypass of inhibited reaction.

B. Chloramphenicol   :   reduced uptake into cell.

C. Tetracycline   : eliminates or reduces binding of antibiotic to cell target enzymatic cleavage or modification to inactivate antibiotic molecule.

D. Erythromycin : eliminates or reduces binding of antibiotic to cell target enzymatic cleavage or modification to inactivate antibiotic molecule.

E. Aminoglycosides : active efflux from the cell.

92   The following are statements regarding tissue specificity of normal flora:

A. Tissue tropism is that the host provides essential nutrients and growth factors for the bacterium.
B. Specific adherence involves biochemical interactions between bacterial surface components and host cell molecular receptors.
C. Majority of normal flora are able to construct biofilms on a tissue surface.
D. Cell-bound protein (M-protein) is used by *Streptococcus pyogenes* in adhesion .
E. Cell-bound protein is used by *Staphylococcus aureus* in adhesion.

93   The following normal bacterial flora are correctly matched with attachment sites of the host:

A. *Streptococcus pyogenes*   : Pharyngeal epithelium.
B. *Staphylococcus aureus*   : Pellicle of tooth.
C. Enterotoxigenic *E. coli*   : Intestinal epithelium.
D. *Treponema pallidum*   : Mucosal epithelium.
E. Mycoplasma   : Respiratory epithelium.

94   The following Predominant normal bacterial flora is correctly matched with anatomical location in adults:

A. Staphylococci   :   Skin.
B. Lactic acid bacteria :   teeth.
C. Streptococci   : pharynx.

D.   Bacteroides   :   colon.

E.   Corynebacteria   :   anterior urethra.

95   The beneficial effects of the normal flora include:

A.   Stimulate the production of vitamins.

B.   Prevent colonization by pathogens by competing for attachment sites or for essential nutrients.

C.   Stimulation of the development of certain tissues,

D.   Antagonize other bacteria through the production of substances which inhibit or kill nonindigenous species.

E.   Stimulate the production of natural antibodies.

96   The harmful effects of the normal flora include:

A.   Bacterial synergism between a member of the normal flora and a potential pathogen.

B.   Competition for nutrients of the host.

C.   Induction of a high grade toxemia.

D.   The normal flora may be agents of disease. Members of the normal flora may cause endogenous disease.

E.   Transfer to susceptible another host.

97   The following are statements regarding disinfection:

A.   It leads to destruction of all pathogenic microbes or their spores.

B.   Moist heat at temperature below 100 degree is used for disinfection of surgical and medical equipments in emergency.

C.   Ultraviolet rays is used to reduce the number of bacteria in air inside operation rooms, laboratory safety cabinet.

D.   High level chemical disinfectants is used for TB bacilli.

E.   Prions is the most resistant organism according to the innate resistance.

98   The following are statements regarding sterilization by heat:

A.   Dry heat is more effective than the moist heat.

B.   Red heat is used for sterilization of the bacteriological loop by heating in the Bunsen flame.

C.   Hot air oven is used for glass ware, and metallic instruments.

D.   Incineration is used for destruction of contaminated materials in the incinerator.

E.   Autoclave is used for sterilization of cotton and gauze.

99   The following are statements regarding disinfectant Selection:

A.   Should be slow acting in presence of organic substances.

B.   Be effective against all types of infectious agents without destroying tissue or acting as a poison if ingested.

C.   Easily penetrate material to be disinfected, without damaging/discoloring it.

D.   Be easy to prepare, stable when exposed to light, heat or other environ-mental factors.

E.   Not have an unpleasant odor.

100   The routine laboratory examinations are useful for bacteriological testing of water include

A.   Presumptive coliform count.

B.   Eijkman test.

C.   Sweep plate method.

D.   Plate count.
E.   Whey agglutination test.

1.2 Questions with answers: (True/False Questions):

1.   Robert Koch:

T   A.   discovered that injected pure cultures of anthrax bacilli into mice and caused anthrax.
T   B.   investigated the aetiology of tuberculosis.
F   C.   developed the first antibiotic that selectively killed the pathogen.
T   D.   formulated Koch's postulates.
F   E.   introduced antiseptic surgery.

2.   Discoveries of Louis Pasteur included:

T   A.   Microorganisms are the causes of infectious disease.
T   B.   Technique of pasteurization.
F   C.   Vaccine against anthrax.
F   D.   Penicillin.
F   E.   Microscope.

3.   Therapeutics include:

T   A.   Drugs.
T   B.   Surgery.
T   C.   Radiation therapy.
F   D.   Tattooing.

T   E.   Psychiatry.

4.   Plasmids:

T   A.   are small circular extra-chromosomal DNA.
T   B.   sizes vary from 1 to 1,000 kilobase pairs.
F   C.   found in eukaryotes.
T   D.   found in prokaryotes.
F   E.   not associated with mechanism of gene transfer.

5.   Autoclave can be used in sterilization of

F   A.   laboratory glassware.
T   B.   surgical instruments.
F   C.   paraffin.
F   D.   powders.
T   E.   rubber gloves.

6.   Bacteria

F   A.   are single- cell eukaryotes.
F   B.   have true nucleus.
T   C.   have rigid cell wall containing peptidoglycan.
T   D.   are classified according to shape, gram staining reaction, oxygen requirement.
T   E.   can grow on inanimate culture medium.

7.   The characteristics of bacteria include:

T   A.   being haploid.

T B. division by binary fission.
F C. having no nuclear membrane.
F D. multicellular eukaryotes with no rigid cell wall.
T E. unicellular organisms with prokaryotic cell structures.

8. Spore forming bacteria are

T A. *Clostridium difficile.*
F B. *Corynebacterium diptheriae.*
T C. *Bacillus anthracis.*
T D. *Clostridium tetani.*
T E. *Bacillus cereus.*

9. Regarding structure of bacteria, the following means:

T A. Spherical or oval = cocci.
F B. rod-shaped = vibrios.
T C. flexous, spiral = spirochaetes.
F D. comma-shaped = actinomycetes.
F E. helical & cylindrical = bacilli.

10 For cultivation of bacteria, the followings should be considered:

T A. choosing appropriate specimen to examine.
T B. specimen should avoid contamination from normal flora.
T C. prompt transportation of the specimen to the laboratory.
T D. essential information about antibiotic.
F E. none of the above.

11 The following statements are true for bacteria:

T   A.   They possess rigid cell wall.

F   B.   They are motile by means of pseudopodia.

F   C.   They cannot be grown on artificial media.

T   D.   They multiply by binary division.

F   E.   Almost all bacteria can form spore.

12   Bacteria that can grow either in the presence or absence of oxygen are called:

T   A.   Facultative anaerobes.

F   B.   Microaerophiles.

F   C.   Strict anaerobes.

F   D.   Obligate aerobes.

F   E.   Obligate anaerobes.

13   Sodium hypochlorite is

F   A.   used for viral environmental disinfection.

T   B.   used on smooth and hard surfaces of the floor.

F   C.   not a useful disinfectant for laboratory discard jars.

T   D.   caustic to the skin at high concentration.

T   E.   an effective disinfectant for *Mycobacterium tuberculosis*.

14   The virulence of the organisms is determined by

F   A.   presence of fimbriae.

F   B.   presence of metachromatic granules.

T   C.   production of toxin.

T   D.   presence of spores.

T   E.   production of aggressive enzymes.

15 Antibiotic resistance among bacteria

T Æ. occurs by altering the number and structure of porins.
T Ʀ. is attributed to plasmids.
F Œ. is estimated by staining techniques.
F Ɖ. is transmitted by virulent bacteriophages.
T E. occurs due to alteration of target sites on the bacteria.

16 The following are statements regarding events of bacterial morphology:

F A. The name spirillum refers to rod-like bacteria.
T B. The name coccus refers to spherical like bacteria.
F C. Bacteria form distinctive cell morphologies when grown on Petri plates.
F D. Bacteria form distinct colony morphologies when examined by light microscopy.
T E. Some bacteria produce elaborate structures bearing reproductive spores (e.g. Myxococcus).

17 The following are statements regarding the primary structure of bacterial biological macromolecules:

T A. The sequence in which the subunits are put together in the macromolecule is called the primary structure.
T B. Primary structure determines many of the properties that the macromolecule will have.
F C. Majority of amino acids of proteins are found in membranes.
T D. Carbohydrates of polysaccharides are found in capsules, inclusions (storage) and cell walls.

T   E.   tRNA is found in cytoplasm.

18   The following are statements regarding bacterial cell wall:

T   A.   It provides structural integrity to the bacterial cell.

T   B.   Peptidoglycan is responsible for the determination of cell shape.

T   C.   Several antibiotics stop bacterial infections by interfering with cell wall synthesis.

T   D.   For both Gram-positive and Gram-negative bacteria, particles of approximately 2 nm can pass through the peptidoglycan.

F   E.   If the bacterial cell wall is entirely removed, it is called a spheroplast.

19   The following are statements regarding bacterial cell wall:

T   A.   It is an essential structure for viability.

F   B.   It is composed of many different components.

T   C.   It is one of the most important sites for attack by antibiotics.

T   D.   It causes symptoms of disease in animals.

T   E.   It provides for immunological distinction and immunological variation among strains of bacteria.

20   The bacterial cell structures are correctly matched with their functions:

T   A.   Cell wall of Gram-positive bacteria : Prevents osmotic lysis of cell protoplast and confers rigidity and shape on cells.

T   B.   Common pilli or fimbriae : protection against phagotrophic engulfment.

T   C.   Plasma membrane   : energy generation and location of numerous enzyme systems.

T   D.   Ribosomes   : Sites of translation (protein synthesis)

T   E.   Plasmid   : Extrachromosomal genetic material.

21   The following major elements are correctly matched with general physiological functions :

T   A.   Oxygen   : Constituent of cell material.

T   B.   Carbon   : Main constituent of cellular material.

T   C.   Nitrogen   : Constituent of amino acids, nucleic acids nucleotides, and coenzymes.

T   D.   Hydrogen   : Main constituent of organic compounds and cell water.

F   E.   Iron :   Main cellular inorganic cation and cofactor for certain enzymes.

22   The following common vitamins required in the nutrition of certain bacteria are correctly matched with following functions

T   A.   Folic acid   :   required for synthesis of purine bases and methionine.

T   B.   Biotin   : Biosynthetic reactions that require CO_2 fixation.

T   C.   Nicotinic acid : Electron carrier in dehydrogenation reactions.

T   D.   Vitamin K   : Electron transport processes.

F   E.   Thiamine (B_1) : Transfer of methyl groups.

23   The following methods used to measure bacterial growth are correctly matched with their applications

T   A.   Direct microscopic count : Enumeration of bacteria in milk or cellular vaccines.

T B. Viable cell count (colony counts) : Enumeration of bacteria in milk, foods, soil, water, laboratory cultures, etc.

F C. Turbidity measurement : Microbiological assays.

T D. Measurement of dry weight or wet weight of cells or volume of cells after centrifugation : Measurement of total cell yield in cultures.

T E. Measurement of total N or protein : Measurement of total cell yield from very dense cultures.

24 The following are statements regarding methods used to measure bacterial growth:

F A. Direct microscopic count can distinguish living from nonliving cells.

T B. Colony counts are very sensitive if plating conditions are optimal.

F C. Turbidity measurement is slow and destructive.

T D. Measurement of total N or protein is only practical application is in the research laboratory.

T E. Measurement of Biochemical activity Requires a fixed standard to relate chemical activity to cell mass and/or cell numbers.

25 The following method used to measure bacterial growth is correctly matched with its application:

T A. Direct microscopic count : Enumeration of bacteria.

T B. Viable cell count (colony counts) : Enumeration of bacteria

T C. Turbidity measurement : Estimations of large numbers of bacteria in clear liquid media and broths.

T D. Measurement of total N or protein : Measurement of total cell yield from very dense cultures.

T   E.   Measurement of dry weight or wet weight of cells or volume of cells after centrifugation : Measurement of total cell yield in cultures.

26   The following Medium is used in generation for some common bacteria under optimal conditions of growth :

T   A.   Glucose-salts : *Escherichia coli.*

T   B.   Sucrose-salts : *Bacillus megaterium.*

T   C.   Heart infusion broth : *Staphylococcus aureus.*

T   D.   Milk : *Lactobacillus acidophilus* .

F   E.   Mannitol-salts-yeast extract : *Treponema pallidum* .

27   The following are statements regarding bacterial mutants:

T   A.   Mutants in bacteria are mostly biochemical in nature.

T   B.   Auxotrophs are the most important mutants.

T   C.   Chemoauxotrophs are mutants that can't use some nutrient (usually a sugar) that prototrophs can use as food.

T   D.   Drug resistance mutants are usually dominant.

T   E.   Auxotrophs and chemoauxotrophs are usually recessive.

28   The following are statements regarding bacterial sexual processes:

T   A.   Conjugation is a direct transfer of DNA from one bacterial cell to another.

T   B.   Transduction is the use of a bacteriophage to transfer DNA between cells.

T   C.   Transformation is a naked DNA is taken up from the

environment by bacterial cells.

T   D.   In transformation the E. coli cells are made "competent" to be transformed by treatment with calcium ions and heat shock.

F   E.   The transduction is the closest analogue in bacteria to eukaryotic sex.

29   Significance of plasmids include

T   A.   codes for resistance to several antibiotics like Gram-negative bacteria carry plasmids that give resistance to antibiotics such as penicillins..

T   B.   codes for the production of toxins (such as Enterotoxins by *Escherichia coli*)

T   C.   codes for resistance to heavy metals such as Hg.

T   D.   plasmids carry virulence determinant genes. Eg, the plasmid Col V of *Escherichia coli* contains genes for iron sequestering compounds.

T   E.   contains genes coding for enzymes that allow bacteria unique or unusual materials for carbon or energy sources.

30   The physiological mechanisms of antibiotic resistance include

F   A.   activation of the antibiotic by enzymes produced by the bacteria.

T   B.   alteration of target proteins such that the antibiotic doesn't bind or binds with decreased affinity.

T   C.   alteration of the membrane which decreases the permeability of the antibiotic.

T   D.   active efflux of the antibiotic.

T   E.   development of alternate metabolic pathway to bypass the action of antibiotic.

31   The following examples of bacteria are correctly matched with
     a method of adhesion to host cell or tissue surfaces:

T   A.   *Streptococcus pyogenes* :   Protein F.
F   B.   *Streptococcus mutans*:   Cell-bound protein .
T   C.   *Neisseria gonorrhoeae*   :   Type IV pili (N-methylphenyl-
          alanine pili)
T   D.   *Enterotoxigenic E. coli*   :   Type-I fimbriae.
T   E.   Mycoplasma   :   Membrane protein.

32   The following extracellular bacterial proteins invasins are
     correctly matched with types of bacteria:

T   A.   Hyaluronidase :   Streptococci .
F   B.   Phospholipases *:   Clostridium* species   .
T   C.   Coagulase *:   Staphylococcus aureus*   .
T   D.   Lecithinases *:   Clostridium perfringens* .
T   E.   Neuraminidase *:   Vibrio cholerae* .

33   The following are statements regarding comparison between
     properties of bacterial endotoxins and classic exotoxin:

T   A.   Relationship to cell is part of outer membrane in endotoxin
          while it is extracellular in ebdotoxin.
F   B.   Endotoxin is usually denatured by boiling while not in
          exotoxin.
T   C.   Both are antigenic.
F   D.   Both can converted to toxoids.
T   E.   Endotoxins are less potent while exotoxins are relatively high
          potency.

34   The following bacterial exotoxins are correctly with their biological effects:

T   A.   Cholera toxin   :   Activates adenylate cyclase; increased level of intracellular cAMP promote secretion of fluid and electrolytes in intestinal epithelium leading to diarrhea.

T   B.   Diphtheria toxin   :   Inhibits protein synthesis resulting in death of the cells.

F   C.   *E. coli* heat-labile toxin LT   :   Blocks inhibition of adenylate cyclase; increased levels of cAMP affect hormone activity and reduce phagocytic activity.

T   D.   *Pseudomonas* Exotoxin A   :   Inhibits protein synthesis in susceptible cells, resulting in death of the cells.

T   E.   *Staphylococcus aureus* Exfoliatin B   :   Separation of the stratum granulosum of the epidermis, between the living layers and the superficial dead layers.

35   The following pore-forming bacterial toxins are correctly matched with the diseased caused:

T   A.   perfringiolysin O from *Clostridium perfringens* :   gas gangrene.

F   B.   Hemolysin from *Escherichia coli* :   diarrhoea .

T   C.   alpha toxin from *Staphylococcus aureus* : abcesses.

T   D.   streptolysin O from *Streptococcus pyogenes* : strep throat.

T   E.   Leukocidin from Staphylococcus aureus :   pyogenic infections.

36   The followings characteristics are generally present in a Gram-positive bacterium:

T   A.   cytoplasmic lipid membrane.

T   B.   teichoic acids in the cell wall.

T   C.   capsule polysaccharides (only in some species)

T   D.   flagellum(only in some species)

F   E.   the transpeptidase creates a covalent bond directly between peptidoglycan molecules, with no intervening bridge.

37   The following are statements regarding Gram-positive bacteria:

T   A.   They are able to retain the crystal violet stain because of their thick peptidoglycan.

T   B.   Plasma membrane, PG layer and cell wall are three distinct structures.

T   C.   They are amorphous and can change shape, since the outer plasma membrane consists of a dynamic lipid bilayer.

F   D.   The S-layer is attached to directly to the outer membrane.

T   E.   They are bounded by a single unit lipid membrane.

38   The following are statements regarding Gram-negative bacteria:

T   A.   In a Gram stain test, a counterstain (commonly safranin) is added after the crystal violet, coloring all gram-negative bacteria with a red or pink color.

F   B.   They are less resistant than gram-positive bacteria against antibiotics.

T   C.   The pathogenic capability of them is often associated with certain components of cell envelope, in particular, the lipopolysaccaride.

T   D.   Gram-negative bacteria associated with nosocomial infections.

T   E.   The proteobacteria are a major group of them.

39   The following characteristics are generally present in a Gram-negative bacteria:

F   A.   Thick peptidoglycan layer.

T   B.   Outer membrane containing lipopolysaccharide.

T   C.   There is a space between the layers of peptidoglycan and the secondary cell membrane called the periplasmic space.

T   D.   The S-layer is directly attached to the outer membrane, rather than the peptidoglycan.

T   E.   No teichoic acids.

40

Gram-negative Bacteria vs Gram-positive Bacteria

		Gram-negative Bacteria	**Gram-positive Bacteria**
T	A.	Peptidoglycan layer is thin.	Peptidoglycan layer is thick.
F	B.	Outer membrane is absent.	Outer membrane is present.
T	C.	Lipid and lipoprotein content is high.	Lipid and lipoprotein content is low.
T	D.	Toxins produced is primarily endotoxins.	Toxins produced is primarily extotoxin
T	E.	More resistance to antibiotics.	More susceptible to antibiotics.

41   The following are statements regarding virulence factors of *S. aureus*:

T   A.   Surface proteins promote colonization of host tissues.

T   B.   Invasins promote bacterial spread in tissues.

F   C.   Surface factors damage host tissues or provoke symptoms of disease.

T   D.   Biochemical properties enhance their survival in phagocytes.

T   E.   Membrane-damaging toxins lyse eucaryotic cell membranes.

42   The following are statements regarding *Streptococcus pyogenes* (Group A streptococcus):

F   A.   It is a Gram-negative bacteria.

T   B.   The metabolism of S. pyogenes is fermentative.

T   C.   It requires enriched medium containing blood in order to grow.

T   D.   Group A streptococci typically have a capsule composed of hyaluronic acid and exhibit beta (clear) hemolysis on blood agar.

T   E.   M protein is a virulence factor of it.

43   The following are statements regarding *Escherichia coli*:

T   A.   It is facultatively anaerobic Gram-negative rods.

F   B.   It can grow in media with glucose and additional growth factors.

T   C.   It is a consistent inhabitant of the human intestinal tract.

T   D.   P fimbriae are used in adhesion.

T   E.   Pathogenic strains of E. coli are responsible for neonatal meningitis.

44   The following are statements regarding diseases caused by *Streptococcus pyogenes*:

T   A.   Suppurative condition occur in the throat.

T   B.   Streptococcal pharyngitis is acquired by inhaling aerosols emitted by infected individuals.

F   C.   Impetigo is the infection of the dermis.

T   D.   Scarlet fever is caused by production of erythrogenic toxin by a few strains of the organism.

T   E.   Toxic shock is caused by a few strains that produce a toxic shock-like toxin.

45   The following are statements regarding *Streptococcus pneumoniae*:

F   A.   It is a normal inhabitant of the human lower respiratory tract.

T   B.   *Streptococcus pneumoniae* cells are Gram-positive, lancet-shaped cocci.

T   C.   They are alpha hemolytic when cultured on blood agar.

T   D.   They do not form spores.

T   E.   It causes osteomyelitis.

46   The following are statements regarding Gram-negative aerobic rods and cocci:

T   A.   This group consists of Gram-negative bacteria phenotypically related to members of the genus *Pseudomonas*.

F   B.   Their metabolism is fermentative.

T   C.   Many bacteria in this group are free-living in soil and water.

T   D.   *Pseudomonas aeruginosa* is a leading cause of hospital-acquired infections.

T   E.   *Bordetella pertussis* causes of Whooping cough.

47   The following are statements regarding Enteric bacteria:

F   A.   They are Gram-positive rods with facultative anaerobic metabolism.

T   B.   This group consists of *Escherichia coli* and its relatives.

T   C.   They all ferment glucose to acid end products.

T   D.   They are consistent members of the normal flora.

T   E.   *Shigella dysenteriae* causes bacillary dysentery.

48   The following are statements regarding *Pyogenic Cocci*:

T   A.   The Gram-positive cocci produce at least a third of all the bacterial infections of humans.

T   B.   *Staphylococcus aureus* occur normally on the nasal membranes.

T   C.   *S. epidermidis* is rarely a pathogen.

F   D.   *S. pyogenes* is coomonly found as normal flora in the upper respiratory tract.

T   E.   *Streptococcus pneumoniae* is the most frequent cause of otitis media.

49   The following are statements regarding Endospore-forming bacteria:

T   A.   They are Gram-positive and usually rod-shaped.

F   B.   *Bacillus anthracis* causes food poisoning.

T   C.   *Clostridium perfringens* causes anaerobic wound infections and gas gangrene.

T   D.   *Clostridium difficile* causes pseudomembranous colitis.

T   E.   *Listeria monocytogenes* does not form endospore.

50   The following are statements regarding vibrios:

T   A.   They are capable of both respiratory and fermentative metabolism.

T   B.   They are distinguished from enterics by being oxidase-positive and motile by means of polar flagella.

T   C.   In liquid media vibrios are motile by polar flagella.

F   D.   *V. parahaemolyticus* is noninvasive, affecting the small intestine through secretion of an enterotoxin.

T   E.   Treatment of cholera involves the rapid intravenous replacement of the lost fluid and ions.

51   The following are statements regarding Salmonella:

T   A.   It is a Gram-negative facultative rod-shaped bacterium.

F   B.   It is the cause of acute gastroenteritis, resulting from bacterial invasion of the bloodstream.

T   C.   All *Salmonella* serovars form a single DNA hybridization group.

T   D.   *Salmonella* typhi produce flagella.

T   E.   Salmonellosis in these cases is transmitted through fecal contamination of water or food.

52   Characteristics of Salmonella include:

F   A.   Gram-positive bacteria.

T   B.   Lactose negative.

T   C.   Methyl red test positive.

T   D.   Citrate positive (growth on Simmon's citrate agar)

T   E.   Urease negative.

53   The following are statements regarding *Pseudomonas aeruginosa*:

T   A.   It is a free-living bacterium.

T   B.   It is primarily a nosocomial pathogen.

T   C.   It causes urinary tract infections.

T   D.   In the laboratory, the simplest medium for growth of *Pseudomonas aeruginosa* consists of acetate as a source of carbon and ammonium sulfate as a source of nitrogen.

F   E.   It is highly sensitive to many antibiotics.

54   The following are statements regarding Shigellae:

F   A.   They are Gram-negative, motile, non-spore forming, rod-shaped bacteria.

T   B.   Eosin methylene blue (EMB) agar is used to determine the bacteria.

T   C.   The primary plating media shown here are, MacConkey agar, ENDO agar, Hektoen enteric (HE) agar and Salmonella-Shigella (SS) agar.

T   D.   *Shigella dysenteriae* type 1, causes deadly epidemics in many developing countries.

T   E.   Ampicillin, is commonly used in treatment.

55   The following are statements regarding Actinobacteria:

T   A.   They are a group of Gram-positive bacteria.

T   B.   They have high guanine and cytosine content in their DNA.

T   C.   Most Actinobacteria of medical significance are in subclass Actinobacteridae, order Actinomycetales.

T   D.   Some Actinobacteria form branching filaments.

F   E.   All actinobacteria are aerobic.

56   The following are statements regarding Mycobacterium:

T   A.   They are aerobic.

T   B.   Mycobacteria do not contain endospores or capsules.

T   C.   They are classified as an acid-fast Gram-positive bacterium.

F   D.   All *Mycobacterium* species have a characteristic thin cell wall.

F   E.   Some species are very easy to culture.

57   The following are statements regarding Mycobacterium:

T   A.   *M. tuberculosis* is nonpigmented in the light and dark.

T   B.   Mycobacteria are classical acid-fast organisms.

T   C.   Stains used in evaluation of tissue specimens or microbiological specimens include Ziehl-Neelsen stain.

T   D.   Mycobacteria appear phenotypically most closely related to members of *Nocardia*, *Rhodococcus* and *Corynebacterium*.

F   E.   All Mycobacteria are found as free-living bacteria.

58   The following are statements regarding anaerobes:

F   A.   They are all Gram-positive.

T   B.   They are commensal organisms of the mouth, oropharynx.

T   C.   Infections with anaerobes are frequently polymicrobial.

T   D.   Often associated with foul or putrid odour.

T   E.   They are usually sensitive to clindamycin.

59   The following are statements regarding anaerobes:

T   A.   They require molecular oxygen as a terminal electron acceptor.

T   B.   Anaerobes cannot grow in the presence of oxygen.

T   C.   Their metabolism is a fermentative type.

T   D.   Many members of the indigenous human flora are anaerobic bacteria.

F   E.   Infections produced by anaerobic bacteria occur in few parts of the human body.

60   The following are statements regarding Spirochaetes:

T   A.   They are chemoheterotrophic in nature.

F   B.   They are distinguished from other bacterial phyla by the type of cell membrane.

T   C.   Most spirochaetes are anaerobic.

T   D.   *Borrelia burgdorferi* causes Lyme disease.

T   E.   *Borrelia recurrentis*, causes relapsing fever .

61   The following are statements regarding Spirochaetes:

F   A.   They are easily observed by light microscope.

T   B.   Most of them appear as helical coils.

T   C.   Their flagella lie between the outer membrane and the peptidoglycan layer,

T   D.   Nonpathogenic treponemes can be found in the oral cavity.

T   E.   Penicillin is used for treatment of all stages of syphilis.

62   The following are statements regarding Chlamydia:

T   A.   Chlamydia infections are the most common leading cause of infectious blindness worldwide.

T   B.   The *Chlamydia suis* species is a human pathogen.

T   C.   It is found in the form of an elementary body and a reticulate body.

F   D.   Commonly Chlamydia infections cause symptoms.

T   E.   Chlamydia is detected by fluorescent monoclonal antibody test.

63   The following are statements regarding Mycoplasma:

F   A.   They are affected by many common antibiotics such as penicillin.

T   B.   They can survive without oxygen.

T   C.   Most of them are pseudococcoidal.

T   D.   They are most require sterols for the stability of their cytoplasmic membrane.

T   E.   *M. pneumoniae* is a cause of atypical pneumonia.

64   The following are statements regarding *Mycoplasma*:

T   A.   *Mycoplasma* species are often found in research laboratories as contaminants in cell culture.

F   B.   They are easily detected by conventional microscope.

T   C.   Mycoplasmas may induce cellular changes, including chromosome aberrations.

T   D.   Enzyme immunoassays is used in their detection.

F   E.   Majority of mycoplasma infections in humans are associated with skin eruptions.

65   The following are statements regarding *Ureaplasma urealyticum*:

T   A.   It is a bacterium belonging to the family Mycoplasmataceae.

T   B.   It is part of the normal genital flora of both men and women.

T   C.   It has been noted as one of the infectious causes of sterile pyuria.

T   D.   Cholesterol is required for their growth.

F   E.   Penicillin is the drug of choice.

66   The following are statements regarding Rickettsias:

T   A.   They are Gram-negative.

T   B.   They divide by binary fission and they metabolize host-derived glutamate.

F   C.   They can grow outside of a host cell.

T   D.   They occur in nature in the gut lining of arthropods.

F   E.   *Rickettsia rickettsii* is the cause of epidemic typhus.

67   The following are statements regarding virulence of Rickettsiae:

T   A.   Rickettsiae are inoculated into the dermis of the skin by a tick bite or through damaged skin from the feces of lice or fleas.

T   B.   The bacteria spread through the bloodstream and infect the endothelium.

T   C.   The adhesins are presumed to be outer membrane proteins.

T   D.   Typhus group rickettsiae are released from host cells by lysis of the cells.

F   E.   Spotted fever group rickettsiae accumulate in large numbers and do lyse the host cells.

68   The following are statements regarding *Orientia tsutsugamushi*:

T   A.   It is the causative organism of scrub typhus.

T   B.   Trombiculid mites is the natural vector and reservoir.

F   C.   Its envelope is similar to that of Gram positive bacteria.

T   D.   It is an obligatory intracellular organism.

T   E.   It is sensitive to doxycycline.

69   The following are statements regarding Ehrlichia:

T   A.   They are transmitted by ticks.

T   B.   They are obligately intracellular pathogens.

F   C.   They infect and kill red blood cells.

T   D.   Onset of its symptoms began exactly 14 days after bite occurred.

F   E.   Penicillin is the drug of choice.

70   The following are statements regarding *Bartonella*:

T   A.   *Bartonella* species are considered as opportunistic pathogens.

T   B.   Mammals are the reservoir hosts.

T   C.   Homeless IV drug users are at high risk for *Bartonella* infections.

T   D.   *Bartonella henselae* is the organism responsible for cat scratch disease.

F   E.   *B. henselae* is generally susceptible to penicillin.

71   The following are statements regarding *Coxiella burnetii*:

T   A.   It is the causative agent of Q fever.

F   B.   It is susceptible to environmental stresses like uv light.

T   C.   Inhalation of one organism will yield disease in 50% of the population.

F   D.   Disease occurs as one stage of respiratory symptoms.

T   E.   A combination of erythromycin and rifampin is highly effective in treatment.

72 *Staphylococci*

F   A.   are catalase test negative.

T   B.   are resistant to bacitracin.

T   C.   are soil microbial flora.

F   D.   do not grow in Mannitol salt agar.

T   E.   grow in a 6.5% NaCl solution.

73 **Spore forming bacteria include**

F   A.   *Haemophilus influenza.*

T   B.   *Bacillus cereus.*

T   C.   *Clostridiumdifficile.*

F   D.   *Corynebacterium diphtheriae.*

F   E.   *Rickettsia prowazekii.*

74 **The pathogenic conditions caused by *Klebsiella pneumoniae* include**

F   A.   pyogenic skin infections.

T   B.   pneumonia .

F   C.   scarlet fever.

T   D.   urinary tract infection.

T   E.   wound infections.

75 *Clostridium difficile*

T   A.   causes nosocomial diarrhoea.

F   B.   infection is treated by amphotericin B.

F   C.   is a gram negative bacilli.

T   D.   is acquired by persons receiving clindamycin in the hospital.

F   E.   is not a primary pathogen for pseudomembranous colitis.

76   *Mycobacterium tuberculosis*

F   A.   causes leprosy in immunocompetent persons.

T   B.   is an acid fast bacillus.

T   C.   is commonly found in patient with HIV infection.

T   D.   is transmitted by inhalation.

F   E.   is treated by single drug therapy.

77   *Mycobacterium leprae*

T   A.   was described by Hansen.

F   B.   can be isolated in artificial culture media.

T   C.   is seen as acid fast bacilli arranged in cigar bundle shape.

T   D.   naturally infects armadillos.

F   E.   causes Lyme disease.

78   *Bacillus anthracis*

T   A.   is a spore-bearing bacilli.

F   B.   causes food poisoning.

T   C.   can be used as a potential biological weapon.

T   D.   infection occurs mainly in humans.

F   E.   is a strict anaerobe.

79   *Pseudomonas aeruginosa*

T   A.   is one of the nosocomial pathogens.

T B. produces blue colored pigments.
T C. can cause wound infection.
F D. is a Gram-positive spore forming bacillus.
F E. can be treated with tetracycline.

80 *Haemophilus influenzae*

T A. is a small gram-negative coccobacillus.
F B. can grow on ordinary culture media.
T C. is responsible for meningitis.
F D. is diagnosed by doing capsule swelling reaction test.
T E. is prevented by the vaccine.

81 The characteristic features of *Mycoplasma pneumoniae* include

T A. obligate intracellular organism.
T B. can cause atypical pneumonia.
F C. transmitted by sexual route.
F D. presence of rigid cell wall.
F E. completely sensitive to penicillin.

82 The virulence factors of *Streptococcus pyogenes* include

T A. lipotechoic acid which facilitates binding to respiratory epithelium.
T B. M-protein which is an adherence protein.
F C. presence of capsule which protects against phagocytosis.
F D. presence of flagella which assist in escaping host defense mechanisms.
T E. production of hyaluronidase which causes spreading cellulitis.

83   The following are statements regarding Lab diagnosis of bacterial infections:

T   A.   *Bacillus anthracis* appear on blood agar as large, grayish, nonhemolytic colonies with irregular borders.

F   B.   Brucella species are diagnosed by culture.

T   C.   *Chlamydia trachomatis* is diagnosed by cellular cytoplasmic inclusions by immunofluorescence technique.

T   D.   *Clostridium botulinum* is diagnosed by culture in standard aerobic culture.

T   E.   *Escherichia coli* (generally) Cultured on MacConkey agar and study carbohydrate fermentation patterns.

84   The following laboratory diagnostic methods are correctly matched with types of bacteria:

T   A.   Culture on Tinsdale agar, followed by immunologic precipitin reaction *Corynebacterium diphtheria*.

T   B.   Culture in 6.5% NaCl   : *Enterococcus faecalis*.

F   C.   Culture on MacConkey agar   :   *Haemophilus influenza*.

T   D.   Urease-positivity   :   *Helicobacter pylori*.

T   E.   Serology for antibodies against O antigen : *Salmonella typhi*.

85   The following are statements regarding microbes that produce natural antibiotics:

T   A.   *Cephalosporium* molds produce the base molecule for development of semisynthetic beta-lactam antibiotics.

T   B.   *Streptomyces* species produce tetracyclines.

T   C.   *Bacillus* species produce polypeptide antibiotics.

T D. The maintenance of a substantial component of the bacterial genome devoted solely to the synthesis of an antibiotic.

F E. Most of the microorganisms that produce antibiotics are sensitive to the action of their own antibiotic.

86 The following are statements regarding characteristics of antibiotics:

T A. Spectrum of action is the range of bacteria or other microorganisms that is affected by a certain antibiotic.

T B. Broad spectrum antibiotics are effective against procaryotes that kill or inhibit a wide range of Gram-positive and Gram-negative bacteria.

T C. Narrow spectrum antibiotics are effective mainly against Gram-positive or Gram-negative bacteria.

T D. Limited spectrum antibiotics are effective against a single organism or disease.

T E. A clinically-useful antibiotic should have a wide spectrum of activity with the ability to destroy or inhibit many pathogenic organisms.

87 A clinically-useful antibiotic should have as many of these characteristics as possible:

T A. It should be without undesirable side effects.

T B. It should be nonallergenic to the host.

T C. It should not eliminate the normal flora of the host.

T D. It should be chemically-stable (have a long shelf-life).

F E. Microbial resistance is common and likely to develop.

88 The following classes of antibiotics are correctly matched with

their spectrum (effective against) :

T   A.   Beta-lactams (penicillins and cephalosporins) :   Gram-positive bacteria.

T   B.   Semisynthetic beta-lactams :   Gram-positive and Gram-negative bacteria.

F   C.   Clavulanic Acid   :   Gram-positive bacteria.

T   D.   Aminoglycosides   :   Gram-positive and Gram-negative bacteria.

T   E.   Lincomycins   :   Gram-positive and Gram-negative bacteria esp. anaerobic *Bacteroides.*

89   The most important targets in bacteria by antibiotic :

T   A.   Bacterial cell wall synthesis.

T   B.   Interfere with protein synthesis.

T   C.   Interference with nucleic acid synthesis.

T   D.   Inhibition of an essential metabolic pathway that exists in the bacterium.

F   E.   Membrane inhibition or disruption works too well.

90   The following are statements regarding MRSA (methicillin/oxacillin-resistant Staphylococcus aureus):

T   A.   It has evolved resistance not only to beta-lactam antibiotics, but to several classes of antibiotics.

T   B.   Some MRSA are resistant to all but one or two antibiotics, notably vancomycin-resistant.

F   C.   Hospital-Associated MRSA (HA-MRSA) occurs less frequently among patients who undergo invasive medical procedures.

T   D.   The main mode of HA-MRSA transmission to other patients is through human hands.

F   E.   Minority of Community-Associated MRSA (CA-MRSA) infections are localized to skin and soft tissue.

91   The following antibiotic is correctly matched with method of resistance:

T   A.   Sulfonamides : metabolic bypass of inhibited reaction.

T   B.   Chloramphenicol   : reduced uptake into cell.

F   C.   Tetracycline   : eliminates or reduces binding of antibiotic to cell target enzymatic cleavage or modification to inactivate antibiotic molecule.

T   D.   Erythromycin : eliminates or reduces binding of antibiotic to cell target enzymatic cleavage or modification to inactivate antibiotic molecule.

F   E.   Aminoglycosides : active efflux from the cell.

92   The following are statements regarding tissue specificity of normal flora:

T   A.   Tissue tropism is that the host provides essential nutrients and growth factors for the bacterium.

T   B.   Specific adherence involves biochemical interactions between bacterial surface components and host cell molecular receptors.

F   C.   Majority of normal flora are able to construct biofilms on a tissue surface.

T   D.   Cell-bound protein (M-protein) is used by *Streptococcus pyogenes* in adhesion.

T   E.   Cell-bound protein is used by *Staphylococcus aureus* in adhesion.

93   The following normal bacterial flora are correctly matched with attachment sites of the host:

T   A.   *Streptococcus pyogenes*   :   Pharyngeal epithelium.

F   B.   *Staphylococcus aureus*   : Pellicle of tooth.

T   C.   Enterotoxigenic *E. coli*   : Intestinal epithelium.

T   D.   *Treponema pallidum*   :   Mucosal epithelium.

T   E.   Mycoplasma   :   Respiratory epithelium.

94   The following Predominant normal bacterial flora is correctly matched with anatomical location in adults:

T   A.   Staphylococci   :   Skin.

F   B.   Lactic acid bacteria :   teeth.

T   C.   Streptococci   :   pharynx.

T   D.   Bacteroides   :   colon.

T   E.   Corynebacteria   : anterior urethra.

95   The beneficial effects of the normal flora include:

F   A.   Stimulate the production of vitamins.

T   B.   Prevent colonization by pathogens by competing for attachment sites or for essential nutrients.

T   C.   Stimulation of the development of certain tissues,

T   D.   Antagonize other bacteria through the production of substances which inhibit or kill nonindigenous species.

T   E.   Stimulate the production of natural antibodies.

96   The harmful effects of the normal flora include:

T   A.   Bacterial synergism between a member of the normal flora and a potential pathogen.

T   B.   Competition for nutrients of the host.

F   C.   Induction of a high grade toxemia.

T   D.   The normal flora may be agents of disease. Members of the normal flora may cause endogenous disease.

T   E.   Transfer to susceptible another host.

97   The following are statements regarding disinfection:

F   A.   It leads to destruction of all pathogenic microbes or their spores.

F   B.   Moist heat at temperature below 100 degree is used for disinfection of surgical and medical equipments in emergency.

T   C.   Ultraviolet rays is used to reduce the number of bacteria in air inside operation rooms, laboratory safety cabinet.

T   D.   High level chemical disinfectants is used for TB bacilli.

T   E.   Prions is the most resistant organism according to the innate resistance.

98   The following are statements regarding sterilization by heat:

F   A.   Dry heat is more effective than the moist heat.

T   B.   Red heat is used for sterilization of the bacteriological loop by heating in the Bunsen flame.

T   C.   Hot air oven is used for glass ware, and metallic instruments.

T   D.   Incineration is used for destruction of contaminated materials in the incinerator.

T   E.   Autoclave is used for sterilization of cotton and gauze.

99   The following are statements regarding disinfectant Selection:

F   A.   Should be slow acting in presence of organic substances.
T   B.   Be effective against all types of infectious agents without destroying tissue or acting as a poison if ingested.
T   C.   Easily penetrate material to be disinfected, without damaging/discoloring it.
T   D.   Be easy to prepare, stable when exposed to light, heat or other environ-mental factors.
T   E.   Not have an unpleasant odor.

100   The routine laboratory examinations are useful for bacteriological testing of water include

T   A.   Presumptive coliform count.
T   B.   Eijkman test.
F   C.   Sweep plate method.
T   D.   Plate count.
F   E.   Whey agglutination test.

2 VIROLOGY

2.1 Questions without answers: (True/False Questions) :

101   The following are statements regarding viruses:

    A.   They replicate only inside the living cells of other organisms.

    B.   They can infect all types of life forms.

    C.   The genetic material made from either DNA or RNA.

    D.   They possess all such qualities of life.

    E.   Viral infections in animals provoke an immune response that usually eliminates the infecting virus.

102   The following are statements regarding general properties of viruses::

A.   All possess envelopes.
B.   Each contains RNA and DNA.
C.   They are motile by means of endoflagella.
D.   They are strict intracellular parasites.
E.   They have nucleic acid surrounded by viral capsid.

103   The following are statements regarding Viral envelope:

A.   glycoproteins play a role in the processes of virus attachment.
B.   is derived from the host cell membrane during the process of virus budding.
C.   is observed by light microscope.
D.   is present in all viruses.
E.   is resistant to ether.

104   The following are statements regarding viral structure:

A.   Most viruses can be seen with an optical microscope.
B.   A virion, consists of nucleic acid surrounded by a protective coat of protein called a capsid.
C.   Viruses can have a lipid "envelope" derived from the host cell membrane.
D.   Nucleocapsid is the association of viral capsid proteins with viral nucleic acid.
E.   Nucleoproteins are proteins associated with nucleic acid.

105   The following are statements regarding viral structure:

A.   A helical structure viruses are composed of a single type of capsomer stacked around a central axis.

B.   The length of a helical capsid is related to the length of the
      nucleic acid contained within it.

C.   Most animal viruses are helical structure viruses.

D.   Prolate structure virus is composed of a cylinder with a cap
      at either end.

E.   Some species of virus envelop themselves in a modified
      form of one of the cell membranes.

106   The following are statements regarding viral genomes:

A.   Viruses as a group, they contain more structural genomic
      diversity than plants and animals.

B.   The vast majority of viruses have RNA genomes.

C.   They are circular, as in the adenoviruses.

D.   The type of nucleic acid is irrelevant to the shape of the
      genome.

E.   A viral genome, irrespective of nucleic acid type, is almost
      always either single-stranded or double-stranded.

107   The following are statements regarding viral genomes:

A.   DNA viruses have smaller genome sizes than RNA
      viruses.

B.   For most viruses with RNA genomes are with single-
      stranded DNA genomes,

C.   Positive-sense viral RNA is in the same sense as viral
      mRNA.

D.   DNA nomenclature for viruses with single-sense genomic
      ssDNA is similar to RNA nomenclature.

E.   Genetic recombination is the process by which a strand of
      DNA is broken and then joined to the end of a different

DNA molecule.

108   The following are statements regarding viral Replication cycle:

A.   Viral populations grow through cell division.

B.   Attachment is a specific binding between viral capsid proteins and specific receptors on the host cellular surface.

C.   Virions enter the host cell through receptor-mediated endocytosis.

D.   Releasing of the viral genomic nucleic acid is the end-result of Uncoating stage.

E.   Replication involves synthesis of viral messenger RNA (mRNA).

109   The following viral classification groups are correctly with its virus example:

A.   dsDNA viruses :   Herpesviruses.

B.   ssDNA viruses (+ strand or "sense") DNA: Poxviruses .

C.   dsRNA viruses :   Reoviruses.

D.   (+)ssRNA viruses (+ strand or sense) RNA :   Picornaviruses.

E.   ssRNA-RT viruses (+ strand or sense) RNA with DNA intermediate in life-cycle   :   Retroviruses.

110   The following are statements regarding RNA viruses:

A.   Replication usually takes place in the cell's nucleus.

B.   Positive-sense viral RNA is similar to mRNA and thus can be immediately translated by the host cell.

C. Rotaviruses is related to double-stranded RNA viruses

D. RNA viruses generally have very high mutation rates compared to DNA viruses.

E. Hepatitis C disease is caused by RNA viruses.

111 The following are statements regarding RNA viruses:

A. Double-stranded RNA viruses (Group III) contain from one to a dozen different RNA molecules.

B. Positive-sense ssRNA viruses (Group IV) have their genome directly utilized as if it were mRNA, with host ribosomes translating it into a single protein.

C. Negative-sense ssRNA viruses (Group V) must have their genome copied by an RNA-dependent RNA polymerase to form positive-sense RNA.

D. Retroviruses (Group VI) have a double-stranded RNA genome.

E. The dsRNA viruses are not closely related to each other.

112 The following are statements regarding DNA viruses:

A. The nucleic acid is usually single-stranded DNA.

B. All three families in the order *Herpesvirales* are double-stranded DNA viruses.

C. Type I genomes are characterized by a small circular DNA genome.

D. Type IV genomes have the largest genomes.

E. All viruses in this group require formation of a replicative form.

113   The following are statements regarding DNA viruses:

A.   The genome replication of most DNA viruses takes place in the cell's nucleus.

B.   The viruses enter the cell by direct fusion with the cell membrane.

C.   Most DNA viruses are entirely dependent on the host cells.

D.   Viruses with a DNA genome can cause cancer.

E.   Small DNA tumor viruses are a group of single-stranded DNA viruses.

114   The following are statements regarding Oncogenic viruses:

A.   The vast majority of human and animal viruses do not cause cancer.

B.   Tumor viruses cause little or no disease after infection in their hosts.

C.   Papilloma viruses are carcinogenic when they integrate into the host cell genome as part of a biological accident.

D.   Human papilloma virus causes transformation in cells through interfering with tumor suppressor proteins.

E.   Merkel cell polyomavirus – a polyoma virus – is associated with the development of Merkel cell carcinoma.

115   The following viruses are correctly matched with type of cancers:

A.   Hepatitis viruses, including hepatitis B and hepatitis C : Hepatocellular carcinoma.

B.   Epstein–Barr virus :   Burkitt's lymphoma.

C.   Merkel cell polyomavirus :   Merkel cell carcinoma.

D.   Kaposi's sarcoma-associated herpesvirus :   primary

effusion lymphoma.

E.   Human T-lymphotropic virus : Cancers of cervix.

116   The following are statements regarding pathogenecity of viral infections:

A.   Most virus infections eventually result in the death of the host cell.

B.   Virus causes cell lysis.

C.   All viruses cause apparent changes to the infected cell.

D.   Cells in which the virus is latent often function normally.

E.   Epstein-Barr virus cause cells to proliferate without causing malignancy.

117   The following are statements regarding innate immunity in viral infections:

A.   Viral replication slowly stimulates innate immunity.

B.   Interferons (IFN) are antiviral factors expressed by many cells when virally infected.

C.   Natural Killer (NK) cells recognize virally infected cells and killthem via cytotoxicity.

D.   Complement proteins MAC can disrupt the viral envelope – Phospholipid bilayer stolen from the host cell.

E.   Complement can opsonize viral particles for phagocytosis.

118   The following are statements regarding role of natural killer (NK) cells in viral infections:

A.   The virally induced MHC class I downregulation triggers NK cells to kill the infected cells.

B.   Recognize infected cells coated with antiviral antibodies using Fc receptors (FcR).

C.. Kill infected cells through antibody dependent cell mediated cytotoxicity (ADCC).

D Produce increased amounts of IFN-δ.

E. Inhibits synthesis of viral proteins.

119   The following are statements regarding acquired immunity in viral infections:

A. Antibodies directed at viral surface antigens are less effective in controlling viral infections.

B. Virus can escape antibody binding by mutating the viral antigen gene.

C. Antibodies can prevent a viral ligand from binding to the host cell receptor and entering the host cell.

D. The antibody can recognize viral antigens on the membrane of the infected cell.

E. Cell is lysed through activation of complement or by ADCC by activating NK cells expressing FcR.

120   Virus infections are confirmed by following diagnostic methods:

A. Detection of virus-specific antibodies in the blood.

B. Detection of virus antigens.

C. Observation of virus particles by fluoresecent microscopy.

D.. Hemagglutination assay.

E. Growth of the virus in a cell culture from a specimen taken from the patient.

121   The following are statements regarding Laboratory diagnosis

of viral infections:

A. In cell culture, the morphologic changes are not specific for the type of virus involved.

B. The presence of IgM in the blood of the host is used to test for an infection sometime in the past.

C. Detection of virus antigens can be done by immunofluorescene technique.

D.
    In hemagglutination assay a viral suspension binds together the red blood cells.

E. Detection of virus encoded DNA and RNA is done with polymerase chain reaction.

122 *Herpes simplex* viruses are

A. able to establish lifelong persistent infections.

B. double stranded RNA viruses.

C. inoculated on Loeffler's serum slope.

D. known to be reactivated by emotional disturbances.

E. susceptible to ampicillin.

123 Epstein-Barr virus is associated with

A. Burkitt's lymphoma.

B. herpes genitalis.

C. Kaposi's sarcoma.

D. nasopharyngeal carcinoma.

E. Shingles.

124 The following are statements regarding Measles and mumps

viruses:

A. A. are transmitted by ingestion of contaminated food.

B. B. belong to *Paramyxoviridae*.

C. C. have one serotype.

D. D. in infections are prevented by MMR vaccine.

E.   infections are confined to humans.

125 Herpes simplex virus type 2 is associated with

A.A. Burkitt's lymphoma.

B.B. herpes genitalis.

C.C. Kaposi's sarcoma.

D.D. nasopharyngeal carcinoma.

E.   small pox.

126 The following are statements regarding Human herpes virus-6:

A.   causes infectious mononucleosis-like illness.

B.   infection is treated by metronidazole.

C.   is a double-stranded DNA virus.

D.   is associated with chicken pox.

E.   is not an oncogenic virus.

127 Flavi viruses include

AA. dengue viruses.

B.   *Herpes simplex* virus.

CC. Japanese encephalitis virus.

DD. *Varicella zoster* virus.

E.   yellow fever virus.

128   The following are statements regarding Influenza A virus:

A.   belongs to family *Orthomyxoviridae*.
BB.   exhibits antigenic drift and antigenic shift.
CC.   gives rise to human influenza pandemics.
DD.   is less virulent than influenza B virus.
E.   is treated by broad spectrum antibiotics.

129   Clinical features of measles include

A.A. bleeding nose.
B.B. conjunctivitis.
C.C. Koplik's spots.
D.D. maculopapular rash.
E.   parotid swelling.

130   The following are statements regarding viral hepatitis (VH):

A.   VHB is one of the blood borne infections.
B.   VHB is considered infectious if levels of HBeAg is high.
C.   VHA runs a chronic course in a majority.
D.   VHD occurs as a co-infection with Hepatitis E.
E.   HVC is best prevented by vaccination.

131   The dengue fever is caused by

A.   Echo virus.

B. Arbo virus.

C. Rhino virus.

D. Orthomyxo virus.

E. Paramyxovirus.

132 The vaccine which successfully prevented to viral infection are

A. Smallpox vaccine.

B. Herpes vaccine.

C. Dengue vaccine.

D. Measle vaccine.

E. Polio vaccine.

2.2 Questions with answers: (True/False Questions) :

101 The following are statements regarding viruses:

T   A.   They replicate only inside the living cells of other organisms.

T   B.   They can infect all types of life forms.

T   C.   The genetic material made from either DNA or RNA.

F   D.   They possess all such qualities of life.

T   E.   Viral infections in animals provoke an immune response that usually eliminates the infecting virus.

102   The following are statements regarding general properties of viruses::

F   A.   All possess envelopes.

F   B.   Each contains RNA and DNA.

F   C.   They are motile by means of endoflagella.

T   D.   They are strict intracellular parasites.

T   E.   They have nucleic acid surrounded by viral capsid.

103   The following are statements regarding Viral envelope:

T   A.   glycoproteins play a role in the processes of virus attachment.

T   B.   is derived from the host cell membrane during the process of virus budding.

F   C.   is observed by light microscope.

F   D.   is present in all viruses.

F   E.   is resistant to ether.

104   The following are statements regarding viral structure:

F   A.   Most viruses can be seen with an optical microscope.

T   B.   A virion, consists of nucleic acid surrounded by a protective coat of protein called a capsid.

T   C.   Viruses can have a lipid "envelope" derived from the host cell membrane.

T   D.   Nucleocapsid is the association of viral capsid proteins with viral nucleic acid.

T   E.   Nucleoproteins are proteins associated with nucleic acid.

105   The following are statements regarding viral structure:

T   A.   A helical structure viruses are composed of a single type of capsomer stacked around a central axis.

T   B.   The length of a helical capsid is related to the length of the nucleic acid contained within it.

F   C.   Most animal viruses are helical structure viruses.

T   D.   Prolate structure virus is composed of a cylinder with a cap at either end.

T   E.   Some species of virus envelop themselves in a modified form of one of the cell membranes.

106   The following are statements regarding viral genomes:

T   A.   Viruses as a group, they contain more structural genomic diversity than plants and animals.

T   B.   The vast majority of viruses have RNA genomes.

F   C.   They are circular, as in the adenoviruses.

T   D.   The type of nucleic acid is irrelevant to the shape of the genome.

T   E.   A viral genome, irrespective of nucleic acid type, is almost always either single-stranded or double-stranded.

107   The following are statements regarding viral genomes:

F   A.   DNA viruses have smaller genome sizes than RNA

viruses.

T   B.   For most viruses with RNA genomes are with single-stranded DNA genomes,

T   C.   Positive-sense viral RNA is in the same sense as viral mRNA.

T   D.   DNA nomenclature for viruses with single-sense genomic ssDNA is similar to RNA nomenclature.

T   E.   Genetic recombination is the process by which a strand of DNA is broken and then joined to the end of a different DNA molecule.

108   The following are statements regarding viral Replication cycle:

F   A.   Viral populations grow through cell division.

T   B.   Attachment is a specific binding between viral capsid proteins and specific receptors on the host cellular surface.

T   C.   Virions enter the host cell through receptor-mediated endocytosis.

T   D.   Releasing of the viral genomic nucleic acid is the end-result of Uncoating stage.

T   E.   Replication involves synthesis of viral messenger RNA (mRNA).

109   The following viral classification groups are correctly with its virus example:

T   A.   dsDNA viruses :   Herpesviruses.

F   B.   ssDNA viruses (+ strand or "sense") DNA: Poxviruses .

T   C.   dsRNA viruses : Reoviruses.

T   D.   (+)ssRNA viruses (+ strand or sense) RNA : Picornaviruses.

T   E.   ssRNA-RT viruses (+ strand or sense) RNA with DNA intermediate in life-cycle : Retroviruses.

110   The following are statements regarding RNA viruses:

F   A.   Replication usually takes place in the cell's nucleus.

T   B.   Positive-sense viral RNA is similar to mRNA and thus can be immediately translated by the host cell.

T   C.   Rotaviruses is related to double-stranded RNA viruses

T   D.   RNA viruses generally have very high mutation rates compared to DNA viruses.

T   E.   Hepatitis C disease is caused by RNA viruses.

111   The following are statements regarding RNA viruses:

T   A.   Double-stranded RNA viruses (Group III) contain from one to a dozen different RNA molecules.

T   B.   Positive-sense ssRNA viruses (Group IV) have their genome directly utilized as if it were mRNA, with host ribosomes translating it into a single protein.

T   C.   Negative-sense ssRNA viruses (Group V) must have their genome copied by an RNA-dependent RNA polymerase to form positive-sense RNA.

F   D.   Retroviruses (Group VI) have a double-stranded RNA genome.

T   E.   The dsRNA viruses are not closely related to each other.

112   The following are statements regarding DNA viruses:

F   A.   The nucleic acid is usually single-stranded DNA.

T   B.   All three families in the order *Herpesvirales* are double
         -stranded DNA viruses.

T   C.   Type I genomes are characterized by a small circular DNA
         genome.

T   D.   Type IV genomes have the largest genomes.

T   E.   All viruses in this group require formation of a replicative
         form.

113   The following are statements regarding DNA viruses:

T   A.   The genome replication of most DNA viruses takes place
         in the cell's nucleus.

T   B.   The viruses enter the cell by direct fusion with the cell
         membrane.

T   C.   Most DNA viruses are entirely dependent on the host cells.

T   D.   Viruses with a DNA genome can cause cancer.

F   E.   Small DNA tumor viruses are a group of single-stranded
         DNA viruses.

114   The following are statements regarding Oncogenic viruses:

T   A.   The vast majority of human and animal viruses do not
         cause cancer.

T   B.   Tumor viruses cause little or no disease after infection in
         their hosts.

T   C.   Papilloma viruses are carcinogenic when they integrate
         into the host cell genome as part of a biological accident.

T   D.   Human papilloma virus causes transformation in cells
         through interfering with tumor suppressor proteins.

T   E.   Merkel cell polyomavirus – a polyoma virus – is
         associated with the development of Merkel cell carcinoma.

115   The following viruses are correctly matched with type of cancers:

T   A.   Hepatitis viruses, including hepatitis B and hepatitis C : Hepatocellular carcinoma.

T   B.   Epstein–Barr virus : Burkitt's lymphoma.

T   C.   Merkel cell polyomavirus : Merkel cell carcinoma.

T   D.   Kaposi's sarcoma-associated herpesvirus : primary effusion lymphoma.

F   E.   Human T-lymphotropic virus : Cancers of cervix.

116   The following are statements regarding pathogenecity of viral infections:

T   A.   Most virus infections eventually result in the death of the host cell.

T   B.   Virus causes cell lysis.

F   C.   All viruses cause apparent changes to the infected cell.

T   D.   Cells in which the virus is latent often function normally.

T   E.   Epstein-Barr virus cause cells to proliferate without causing malignancy.

117   The following are statements regarding innate immunity in viral infections:

F   A.   Viral replication slowly stimulates innate immunity.

T   B.   Interferons (IFN) are antiviral factors expressed by many cells when virally infected.

T   C.   Natural Killer (NK) cells recognize virally infected cells and kill them via cytotoxicity.

T   D.   Complement proteins MAC can disrupt the viral envelope – Phospholipid bilayer stolen from the host cell.

T   E.   Complement can opsonize viral particles for phagocytosis.

118   The following are statements regarding role of natural killer (NK) cells in viral infections:

T   A.   The virally induced MHC class I downregulation triggers NK cells to kill the infected cells.

T   B.   Recognize infected cells coated with antiviral antibodies using Fc receptors (FcR).

T   C..   Kill infected cells through antibody dependent cell mediated cytotoxicity (ADCC).

T   D   Produce increased amounts of IFN-δ.

F   E.   Inhibits synthesis of viral proteins.

119   The following are statements regarding acquired immunity in viral infections:

F   A.   Antibodies directed at viral surface antigens are less effective in controlling viral infections.

T   B.   Virus can escape antibody binding by mutating the viral antigen gene.

T   C.   Antibodies can prevent a viral ligand from binding to the host cell receptor and entering the host cell.

T   D.   The antibody can recognize viral antigens on the membrane of the infected cell.

T   E.   Cell is lysed through activation of complement or by ADCC by activating NK cells expressing FcR.

120   Virus infections are confirmed by following diagnostic methods:

T   A.   Detection of virus-specific antibodies in the blood.

T   B.   Detection of virus antigens.

F   C.   Observation of virus particles by fluoresecent microscopy.

T   D.   Hemagglutination assay.

T   E.   Growth of the virus in a cell culture from a specimen taken from the patient.

121   The following are statements regarding Laboratory diagnosis of viral infections:

F   A.   In cell culture, the morphologic changes are not specific for the type of virus involved.

F   B.   The presence of IgM in the blood of the host is used to test for an infection sometime in the past.

T   C.   Detection of virus antigens can be done by immunofluorescene technique.

T   D.

       In hemagglutination assay a viral suspension binds together the red blood cells.

T   E.   Detection of virus encoded DNA and RNA is done with polymerase chain reaction.

122   *Herpes simplex* viruses are

T   A.   able to establish lifelong persistent infections.

F   B.   double stranded RNA viruses.

F   C.   inoculated on Loeffler's serum slope.

T   D.   known to be reactivated by emotional disturbances.

F   E.   susceptible to ampicillin.

123   Epstein-Barr virus is associated with

T   A.   Burkitt's lymphoma.

F   B.   herpes genitalis.

F   C.   Kaposi's sarcoma.

T   D.   nasopharyngeal carcinoma.

F   E.   Shingles.

124   The following are statements regarding Measles and mumps viruses:

F   A.E.   are transmitted by ingestion of contaminated food.

T   B.F.   belong to *Paramyxoviridae*.

T   C.G.   have one serotype.

T   D.H.   in infections are prevented by MMR vaccine.

T   E.   infections are confined to humans.

125   Herpes simplex virus type 2 is associated with

F   A.E.   Burkitt's lymphoma.

T   B.F.   herpes genitalis.

F   C.G.   Kaposi's sarcoma.

F   D.H.   nasopharyngeal carcinoma.

F   E.   small pox.

126   The following are statements regarding Human herpes virus-6:

F   A.   causes infectious mononucleosis-like illness.

F   B.   infection is treated by metronidazole.

T   C.   is a double-stranded DNA virus.

F   D.   is associated with chicken pox.

T   E.   is not an oncogenic virus.

127   Flavi viruses include

T   AE.   dengue viruses.

F   B.   *Herpes simplex* virus.

T   CG.   Japanese encephalitis virus.

F   DH.   *Varicella zoster* virus.

T   E.   yellow fever virus.

128   The following are statements regarding Influenza A virus:

T   A.   belongs to family *Orthomyxoviridae*.

T   B.   exhibits antigenic drift and antigenic shift.

T   CG.   gives rise to human influenza pandemics.

F   DH.   is less virulent than influenza B virus.

F   E.   is treated by broad spectrum antibiotics.

129   Clinical features of measles include

F   A.E.   bleeding nose.

T   B.F.   conjunctivitis.

T   C.G.   Koplik's spots.

T   D.H.   maculopapular rash.

F   E.   parotid swelling.

130   The following are statements regarding viral hepatitis (VH):

T   A.   VHB is one of the blood borne infections.

T   B.   VHB is considered infectious if levels of HBeAg is high.

F   C.   VHA runs a chronic course in a majority.

F   D.   VHD occurs as a co-infection with Hepatitis E.

F   E.   HVC is best prevented by vaccination.

131   The dengue fever is caused by

F   A.   Echo virus.

T   B.   Arbo virus.

F   C.   Rhino virus.

F   D.   Orthomyxo virus.

F   E.   Paramyxovirus.

132   The vaccine which successfully prevented to viral infection are

T   A.   Smallpox vaccine.

F   B.   Herpes vaccine.

F   C.   Dengue vaccine.

T   D.   Measle vaccine.

T   E.   Polio vaccine.

3 MYCOLOGY

3.1 Questions without answers: (True/False questions):

133   The following are statements regarding general properties of fungi:

    A.   They grow in as yeast or/ and mould form.

    B.   Their spores are derived from asexual or sexual reproduction.

    C.   They possess rigid cell wall.

    D.   Most of the fungi prefer alkaline pH for their growth.

    E.   Sterol is present in their cell membrane.

134   The following are statements regarding structure of fungi:

    A.   The single-celled fungus reproduces by simple budding to form blastoconidia.

B.   Colonies of single-celled fungus are usually dry.

C.   Structures of a filamentous or mould form is a vegetative growth of filaments,such as mushrooms.

D.   The filamentous form reproduces by spores or conidia.

E.   A mass of hyphae collectively make up the mycelium.

135   The following are statements regarding pathogenic fungi:

A.   Infections by candida species are difficult to treat and can be very serious.

B.   Allergies and asthma are thought to be caused by an active host immune response against the presence of candida infection.

C.   Aspergillus flavus produces aflatoxin which is both a toxin and a carcinogen.

D.   *Cryptococcus neoformans* can cause a severe form of meningitis and meningo-encephalitis in patients with HIV infection.

E.   Infection by *Histoplasma capsulatum* is usually due to ingestion contaminated food.

136   The following are statements regarding fungal pathogenicity:

A.   Temperature is a minor physiologic barrier to fungal growth within the human body.

B.   Most fungi are saprophytic.

C.   The basic mechanism of fungal pathogenicity is its ability to adapt to the tissue environment.

D.   The development of human mycoses is related primarily to the infecting organism.

E.   Human body has a highly efficient set of cellular defences to combat fungal proliferation.

137   Laboratory specimens used in systemic opportunistic fungal infections are

A.   skin scrapings.
B.   urine.
C.   sputum.
D.   pleural fluid.
E.   tissue biopsy.

138   Laboratory tests used in diagnosis of systemic opportunistic fungal infections are

A.   Direct microscopy.
B.   Histopathology by H&E stain.
C.   Culture and identification.
D.   Haemagglutination test.
E.   serodiagnostic tests.

139   Superficial (cutaneous) fungal infections are caused by

A.   *Coccidioides* species.
B.   *Epidermophyton* species.
C.   *Histoplasma* species.
D.   *Microsporum* species.
E.   *Trichophyton* species

140   Antifungal agents include

A. Acyclovir.
B. Amphotericin B.
C. Griseofulvin.
D. Ketoconazole.
E. Metronidazole

3.2 Questions with answers: (True/False questions) :

133   The following are statements regarding general properties of fungi:

T   A.   They grow in as yeast or/ and mould form.

T   B.   Their spores are derived from asexual or sexual reproduction.

T   C.   They possess rigid cellwall.

F   D.   Most of the fungi prefer alkaline pH for their growth.

F   E.   Sterol is present in their cell membrane.

134   The following are statements regarding structure of fungi:

T   A.   The single-celled fungus reproduces by simple budding to form blastoconidia.

F   B.   Colonies of single-celled fungus are usually dry.

T   C.   Structures of a filamentous or mould form is a vegetative growth of filaments,such as mushrooms.

T   D.   The filamentous form reproduces by spores or conidia.

T   E.   A mass of hyphae collectively make up the mycelium.

135   The following are statements regarding pathogenic fungi:

T   A.   Infections by candida species are difficult to treat and can be very serious.

F   B.   Allergies and asthma are thought to be caused by an active host immune response against the presence of candida infection.

T   C.   Aspergillus flavus produces aflatoxin which is both a toxin and a carcinogen.

T   D.   *Cryptococcus neoformans* can cause a severe form of meningitis and meningo-encephalitis in patients with HIV infection.

F   E.   Infection by *Histoplasma capsulatum* is usually due to ingestion contaminated food.

136   The following are statements regarding fungal pathogenicity:

F   A.   Temperature is a minor physiologic barrier to fungal growth within the human body.

T   B.   Most fungi are saprophytic.

T   C.   The basic mechanism of fungal pathogenicity is its ability to adapt to the tissue environment.

F   D.   The development of human mycoses is related primarily to the infecting organism.

T   E.   Human body has a highly efficient set of cellular defences to combat fungal proliferation.

137   Laboratory specimens used in systemic opportunistic fungal infections are

T   A.   skin scrapings.

T   B.   urine.

T   C.   sputum.

T   D.   pleural fluid.

T   E.   tissue biopsy.

138   Laboratory tests used in diagnosis of systemic opportunistic fungal infections are

T   A.   Direct microscopy.

T   B.   Histopathology by H&E stain.

T   C.   Culture and identification.

F   D.   Haemagglutination test.

T   E.   serodiagnostic tests.

139   Superficial (cutaneous) fungal infections are caused by

F   A.   *Coccidioides* species.

T   B.   *Epidermophyton* species.

F   C.   *Histoplasma* species.

T   D.   *Microsporum* species.

T   E.   *Trichophyton* species

140   Antifungal agents include

F   A.   Acyclovir.

T   B.   Amphotericin B.

T   C.   Griseofulvin.

T   D.   Ketoconazole.

F   E.   Metronidazole

4 CLINICAL & APPLIED MICROBIOLOGY

4.1 Questions without answers: (True/False questions):

141 The following age group is correctly matched with the most common causative microorganism of osteomyelitis:

A. Newborns (younger than 4) : group A and B *Streptococcus* species.
B. Children (aged 4 to 4 y) : *S. aureus*, group A *Streptococcus* species.
C. Children, adolescents (aged 4 y to adult) : *S. aureus* .
D Adult   : *Streptococcus* species.
.
E. Sickle cell anemia patients : *Salmonella* species .

142 The following are statements regarding osteomyelitis (OM):

A. It can be subclassified on the basis of the causative organism.
B. Chronic OM is often defined as OM that has been present for more than one month.
C. Microorganisms may infect bone via the bloodstream.

D. Pus spreads into the bone's blood vessels, impairing their flow, and areas of devitalized infected bone, known as *sequestra*.
E. Involucrum is the area of necrosis.

143 **The following are statements regarding osteomyelitis:**

A. In children, the long bones are usually affected.
B. In adults, the vertebrae and the pelvis are most commonly affected.
C. Acute osteomyelitis almost invariably occurs in children.
D. Osteomyelitis is a secondary complication in majority of patients with pulmonary tuberculosis.
E. In tubercular osteomyelitis, the long bones and vertebrae are the ones that tend to be affected.

144 **The following are statements regarding osteomyelitis:**

A. *Staphylococcus aureus* is the organism most commonly isolated from all forms of osteomyelitis.
B. Bloodstream-sourced osteomyelitis is seen most frequently in adults.
C. *Blastomyces dermatitidis* is the two most common cause of mycotic osteomyelitis.
D. Diagnosis of osteomyelitis is often based on radiologic results showing a lytic center with a ring of sclerosis.
E. Presence of sepsis is commonly complicate osteomyelitis.

145 **The following are statements regarding Brodie abscess:**

A. It is a subacute osteomyelitis, which may persist for years before converting to a frank osteomyelitis.
B. It is a well-defined cavity in cancellous bone
C. Nocturnal localized pain is a clinical presentation.
D. Brodie's abscess is best visualized using X-ray.

E. The treatment of choice is by antibiotics.

146   The following are statements regarding acute septic arthritis:

A. Direct invasion is the route of Infection.
B. Haemophilus influenzae is a causative organism.
C. Acute synovitis with purulent joint effusion is a finding.
D   Blood culture is used in investigation.
.
E. Complete recovery is a sequelae.

147   The following are statements regarding tuberculosis of bone and joint:

A. It is particularly likely to attack the spine and the ends of the long bones.
B. If not treated, the spinal segments may collapse and cause paralysis in one or both legs.
C. Tuberculous granuloma is a finding.
D   Present with abscess or kyphosis.
.
E. Joint aspiration for AAFB identified in majority of patients.

148   The following are statements regarding Viral exanthems:

A. They are more common among adults.
B. In children, they are most often related to infection.
C. Determining the cause of an exanthem is based on the characteristic morphology, distribution and time course of the eruption.
D   Measles is caused by a ssRNA virus belonging to the
.   *Paramyxoviridae* family.
E. The measles's eruption typically resolves in the same order as its appearance.

149   The following are statements regarding Measles:

A. It has an incubation period of approximately 10–12 days.
B. Koplik spots is seen during the prodromal phase.
C. Typical exanthem begins from the 1st day of infection.
D   Transient immunosuppression is a complications.

.
E.   It is treated by antiviral therapy.

150   The following are statements regarding Rubella:

A.   It is caused by an RNA virus in the *Togaviridae* family.
B.   Majority of infected individuals become symptomatic.
C.   A maculopapular exanthem appears after approximately 2–5 days.
D   The diagnosis of rubella can be made with IgM antibody
.   titers.
E.   Congenital rubella syndrome is the most serious complication.

151   The following are statements regarding erythema infectiosum:

A.   It is a common childhood exanthematous illness caused by parvovirus B19.
B.   Patients present with fiery-red facial erythema after incubation period for 3-4 weeks.
C.   The exanthem recurs intermittently in response to stimuli, such as local irritation, high temperatures and emotional stress.
D   An ELISA is commercially available with high sensitivity in
.   diagnosis.
E.   PCR can detect viral DNA in patient's urine.

152   The following are statements regarding Roseola Infantum:

A.   It is caused by human herpesvirus types 6 and 7.
B.   By the end of the second year of life, approximately half of all children are seropositive for HHV-6.
C.   The incubation period is 5–15 day.
D   Roseola infection can cause leukopenia.
.
E.   The diagnosis of roseola is made by laboratory detection of HHV-6 and -7.

153   The following are statements regarding Epstein–Barr Virus

infection:

A. Epstein–Barr virus (EBV) is a member of the *Herpesvirus* family, belonging to the genus *Lymphocryptovirus.*
B. Half of children infected with EBV manifest an exanthema.
C. A characteristic bright-red morbilliform eruption almost always occurs if mpicillin is administered to the infected child.
D. The eruption most likely results from ampicillin–antibody immune complexes as a consequence of polyclonal B-cell activation.
E. This reaction is considered a true drug allergy.

154 The following are statements regarding Varicella & Herpes Zoster:

A. Varicella is caused by varicella-zoster virus (VZV), an enveloped RNA virus.
B. The transmission of virus requires skin-to-skin contact.
C. The virus initially undergoes primary replication, beginning 3–4 days after exposure.
D. The exanthem begins soon after as erythematous pruritic macules.
E. Bacterial superinfection is the most common complication of varicella.

155 The following are statements regarding Eczema Herpeticum:

A. It is a severe form of disseminated cutaneous HSV infection, which occurs primarily in individuals with atopic dermatitis.
B. Defective cytokine secretion in skin appear to play a role in the pathogenesis.
C. Patients present with monomorphic umbilicated vesiclulopustules.
D. The diagnosis is made clinically.
E. Topical steroids is the drug of choice.

156 The following are statements regarding Hand–Foot–Mouth Disease:

A. It is an exanthem caused by viruses of the *Picornaviridae* family in the *Enterovirus* genus.
B. The most common pathogen is the Coxsackie A16 virus.
C. The infection has a typical incubation period of 10-15 days.
D. Appearance of painful oval, gray vesicles is the main manifestation followed by fever and lymphadenopathy.
E. The vesicles are often arranged parallel to the dermatoglyphs.

157 The following are statements regarding papular acrodermatitis of childhood (PAC):

A. It is a unique cutaneous disorder characterized by the abrupt onset of an erythematous papular exanthema.
B. It is primarily affecting children between 8 and 12 years of age.
C. it was believed that PAC is a manifestation of hepatitis A infection.
D. Occasionally, the papules coalesce into larger plaques and become hemorrhagic or form scales.
E. Treatment is by antiviral therapy.

158 The following are statements regarding papular purpuric glove and socks syndrome (PPGSS):

A. It is usually caused by parovovirus B19.
B. Clinically, it is characterized by symmetric, painful erythema, and edema of the hands and feet that later progresses to a petechial rash.
C. Edema and erythema cann't be observed on the buccal and genital mucosa.
D. Patients with PPGSS are contagious when they exhibit the exanthem.
E. Treatment is symptomatic.

159 The following are statements regarding Impetigo:

A. It is always caused by b-hemolytic streptococci and/or *S. aureus*.
B. Its peak incidence is among children aged 10-12 years.
C. It is usually occurs on exposed areas of the body, most

frequently the face and extremities.

D. During the course of 2– 3 weeks, streptococcal strains transferred from the skin lesions to the upper respiratory tract.

E. The anti–streptolysin O response is strong in patients with streptococcal impetigo.

160 The following are statements regarding cutaneous abscesses:

A. *S. aureus* is usually the causative pathogen in majority of cases.

B. The inflammation and purulence occur as infectious complication.

C. High fever is a presentation.

D. Gram stain and culture are commonly uased in diagnosis.

E. Extensive surrounding cellulitis, is a complication.

161 The following are statements regarding furuncles:

A. They are usually caused by *S. aureus.*

B. They differ from folliculitis, in which inflammation is more superficial and pus is present in the epidermis.

C. They occur mainly in hairy scalp.

D. The lesion consists of an inflammatory nodule and an overlying pustule through which hair emerges.

E. Systemic antibiotics are usually necessary in treatment.

162 The following are statements regarding erysipelas:

A. It affects the deeper dermis, as well as subcutaneous fat.

B. It is more common among adults between 20-40 years.

C. It is almost always caused by b-hemolytic streptococci (usually group A).

D. Penicillin is the treatment of choice.

E. The prognosis is excellent.

163   **The following are statements regarding cellulitis:**

A.   It is an acute spreading infection of the skin, extending more deeply than erysipelas to involve the subcutaneous tissues.
B.   It is almost always caused by b-hemolytic streptococci (usually group A).
C.   Rapidly spreading areas of edema is a manifestation.
D.   Systemic manifestations are usually severe.
E.   Blood culture results are positive in majority of cases.

164   **The following are statements regarding necrotizing skin and soft-tissue infections:**

A.   They are often deep and devastating.
B.   They are usually secondary infections.
C.   They are usually monomicrobial (streptococci).
D.   Presence of gas in the soft tissues is a clinical feature.
E.   They require operative intervention.

165   **The following are statements regarding necrotizing fasciitis:**

A.   Insect bite is an initial lesion.
B.   *S. pyogenes* is causative microorganism.
C.   Approximately two-third of cases in the upper extremities.
D.   Diabetes is an underlying cause.
E.   In the polymicrobial form, an average of 5 pathogens different anaerobic and aerobic organisms can be cultured from the involved fascial plane in each wound.

166   **The following are statements regarding anaerobic streptococcal myositis:**

A.   It causes a less indolent infection than other streptococci.
B.   It is usually associated with trauma or a surgical procedure.
C.   Incision and drainage are critical.
D.   Antibiotic treatment is highly effective.

E.   Penicillin or ampicillin should be administered in high doses.

167   The following are statements regarding pyomyositis:

A.   It is caused mainly by *S. aureus.*
B.   Blood culture results are positive in majority of cases.
C.   Localized pain in a single muscle group is a presenting finding.
D   The disease occurs most often in trunk muscles.

E.   Antibiotics plus extensive surgical incision and drainage are required for appropriate management.

168   The following are statements regarding fournier gangrene:

A.   It involves the scrotum and penis or vulva.
B.   The mean age of onset is 30 years.
C.   Most cases are caused by *S. aureus.*
D   Most patients initially have a urinary tract tract.

E.   Aggressive surgical exploration and appropriate debridement is necessary to remove all necrotic tissue.

169   The following are statements regarding clostridial myonecrosis:

A.   *C. novyi* is the most frequent cause of trauma associated gas gangrene.
B.   *C. septicum* is the causative of spontaneous gangrene.
C.   Skin may initially be pale.
D   Gas in the tissue, detected as crepitus.

E.   Tetracycline is the drug of choice.

170   The following are statements regarding anthrax:

A.   The incubation period of 14-20 days.

B.   Regional lymphadenopathy is common presentation.
C.   Blood culture results are almost always negative.
D.   Immunohistochemical staining is useful in diagnosis.
E.   Penicillin is effective therapy.

171   **The following are statements regarding malasseziosis:**

A.   There are Hypo- to hyperpigmented patches with scales.
B.   Can cause folliculitis.
C.   These fungi also cause dandruff.
D.   Presence of sphaghetti and meatballs of oval to round budding yeasts is diagnostic.
E.   It is treated by excessive washing by soap.

172   **The following are statements regarding dermatophytoses:**

A.   *Microsporum* is a cause.
B.   It may acquired from other animals.
C.   Microscopic observation of fungal elements in skin samples is diagnostic.
D.   Human genetics may play a role in making some families more susceptible to some of these fungi.
E.   Corporis type is treated by systemically applied doses of fluconazole.

173   **The following are statements regarding pityriasis versicolor:**

A.   Malassezia furfur is an etiological agent.
B.   An asymtomatic benign infection of the stratum corneum layer of skin.
C.   It is common in cold climate.
D.   Diagnosis commonly require for tissue biopsies.
E.   The confirmatory test is by direct microscopy of skin scrapings mounted in 10% potassium hydroxide.

174   **The following are statements regarding Eumycetoma:**

A. It is a chronic subcutaneous infection that can spread to bone and lymph tissue.
B. Formation of grains (colonies) is characteristic.
C. It is caused by Aerobic actinomycetes.
D. The disease develops typically as a result of a minor trauma that implants the etiological agent.
E. It is self-limited disease.

175 The following are statements regarding chromoblastomycosis:

A. It is a chronic skin fungal infection.
B. Fungal agents are whitely pigmented.
C. Lesions are nodular and verrucous.
D. Infections tend to be of the lower extremities.

E. *Fonsecea pedrosoi* is causative agent.

176 The following are statements regarding *Tinea nigra*:

A. It is a superficial asymtomatic mycosis.
B. It is more common in cold areas.
C. Exophialia (Phaeoanellomyces) wernekii is an etiologic agent.
D. Pigmented macules on palms or/ and soles are presentations.

E. Direct microscopy of skin scrapings mounted in 10% potassium hydroxide is diagnostic.

177 The following are statements regarding mycetoma:

A. It is caused by a wide variety of free-living or exogenous aerobic actinomycetes.
B. It is most prevalent in tropical and subtropical regions.
C. Actinomycotic Mycetoma is presented as red grain.
D. In Eumycotic Mycetoma the organisms appear as fungal hyphae 2-6 or more width.
E. Actinomycotic Mycetoma is treated by Surgical excision or Amputation.

178   The following are statements regarding chromoblastomycosis:

A.   It is chronic, pruritic, progressive, indolent lesion.
B.   It is most common in tropical or subtropical areas especially in bare-footed agriculture workers.
C.   Cladophialophoracarrionii is causative agent.
D.   It is transmitted by person to person spread.
E.   Large papillomatous lesion involving large portion of the limb is a presentation.

179   The following are statements regarding sporotrichosis:

A.   It is chronic cutaneous or systemic mycosis caused by the thermally dimorphic fungus.
B.   It is transmitted by person to person.
C.   It is worldwide in distribution, but most in temperate as well as tropical region.
D.   Cutaneous form consisting of a linear chain of painless subcutaneous nodules.
E.   Systemic form is often localized in a single organ system.

180   The following are statements regarding infections by Aspergillus species:

A.   They occur in majority of patients who have prolonged neutropenia.
B.   *Aspergillus fumigatus* is the most frequently isolated species.
C.   They may occur locally at sites of intravenous catheter insertion.
D.   They produce painful skin nodules.
E.   Skin lesions resemble pyoderma gangrenosum lesions.

181   Risks for CNS infections include

A.   Extremes of age.

B.   Immunocompromised.
C.   Head Trauma.
D   Labrotomy.
.
E.   Chronic alcoholi/cirrhosis.

182   The following CNS infections are correctly matched with their common causative agents:

A.   Bacterial meningitis :   Pneumococcus.
B.   Viral meningitis   : Enteroviruses.
C.   Fungal meningitis   : Cryptococcus.
D   Encephalitis   : Staph aureus.
.
E.   Brain abcess   :   Anerobes.

183   The following are statements regarding viral menigitis:

A.   Age usually is above 40yo.
B.   Photophobia is a presentation.
C.   Enteroviruses are the main causative virus.
D.   Hematogenous spread to CNS is a route of infection.
E.   Normal glucose is a laboratory finding.

184   The following are statements regarding viral encephalitis:

A.   EBV is one of causative agents.
B.   Psychiatric presentations is clue for Herpes zoster etiology.
C.   Arboviruses are the common causative agent among parkinsonism patients.
D.   EEG is normal in viral encephalitis.
E.   MRI is used in diagnosis.

185   The following are statements regarding HSV encephalitis:

A.   Severe neurological defects occur in minority of patients.
B.   Nearly 1/3 of infections are primary infections.
C.   Affection of temporal lobes and frontal lobes produce the

    psychiatric features.

D. Fever is a presentation in majority of patients.

E. High protein is a laboratory finding of CSF.

186 The following are statements regarding viral meningitis:

A. Herpes simplex virus is one of the causative agents.
B. Enteroviruses are the most common causative viruses.
C. More cases occur during the winter months.
D. The inability to isolate bacterial pathogens in relation to viral meninigits has led to the term ''aseptic meningitis.
E. The clinical course of most of types of viral meningitis is sever and lethal.

187 The following are statements regarding viral encephalitis:

A. Rabies one of the causative agents.
B. The arboviruses are transmitted through blood transfusions.
C. Altered levels of consciousness is common clinical feature.
D. Lumpur puncture often shows a picture compatible with aseptic meningitis.
E. Only HSV disease has specific therapy available.

188 The following are statements regarding Prion disease in CNS:

A. It aggregate extracellularly within the central nervous system to form plaques.
B. The lesion is characterized by vacuole formation in the neurons.
C. The incubation period for prion disease is relatively less than one month.
D. The disease progresses rapidly, leading to brain damage and death.
E. Astemizole has been found to have anti prion infection.

189 The following are statements regarding *Prion diseases in CNS*:

A. They are transmissible spongiform encephalopathies.
B. There are human and animal forms.
C. They are rare.
D They cause neurodegeneration.
.
E. They are self-limited diseases.

190 The following are statements regarding bacterial meningitis:

A. Pneumococcus is the most common cause.
B. Mortality 50 - 90% with severe initial neurologic impairment.
C. Bacteria can cross BBB and enter CSF usually at choroid plexi/dural sinuses.
D Decreased CSF protein due to vascular permeability and
. leakage.
E. Meningismus is a presentation in majority of cases.

191 Causal organism of aseptic meningitis include

A. *Staphylococcus aureus.*
B. *Leptospira interrogans.*
C. *Polio virus.*
D. *Treponema pallidum.*
E. *Haemophillus influenzae .*

192 The following are statements regarding investigations findings in bacterial meningitis:

A. Increased wbc in CSF.
B. Decrease glucose in CSF.
C. Increased protein in CSF.
D If Gram stain -ve intracellular diplococci means the cause is
. Pneumococcus.
E. If Gram stain -ve bacilli means the causative agent is Ecoli.

193 The following are statements regarding bacterial meningitis:

A. Neisseria meningitides affect adults more than 45 years of age.

B.   The disease appears to occur in males more than females.

C.   The infectious organism first colonizes the nasopharynx..

D.   Rapid onset of fever is common clinical presentation.

E.   In most patients with bacterial meningitis, lumpur puncture can be safely performed without antecedent neuroimaging.

194   The following are statements regarding brain abscess:

A.   Brain abscess secondary to otitis media occur more frequently among young adults.

B.   Neck rigidity is rare.

C.   Ring-enhancing lesion with surrounding edema is the finding of CT scan.

D.   Lumpur puncture is help in diagnosis.

E.   Treatment is usually includes a third generation cephalosporin and metronidazole.

195   The following are statements regarding Tuberculous meningitis:

A.   Confusion is an early feature.

B.   Majority of patients with miliary TB have TB meningitis.

C.   Analysing of cerebrospinal fluid is diagnostic.

D.   The CSF usually has a high protein and low glucose.

E.   Hydrocephalus is a complication.

196   The following are statements regarding fungal meningitis:

A.   *Cryptococcus neoformans* is the cause.

B.   The infection is by inhalation.

C.   Rapid development of symptoms.

D.   Decreased glucose in CSF.

E.   Amphotericin B + 5-fluorocytosin is the drug of choice.

197 **The following predisposing factors are correctly matched with the specific pathogen:**

A. Neonatal age : *E.coli.*
B. Otitis media and sinusitis : *S.pneumoniae.*
C. Penetrating head trauma or neurosurgery : *S.aureus.*
D. immunocompromised host : *Mycobacterium tuberculosis.*

E. Endocarditis : *S.aureus.*

198 **The following are statements regarding nosocomial infection:**

A. It is a clinical infection that was neither present nor was in its incubation period when the patient entered the hospital.
B. Must make their appearance before discharge from the hospital.
C. Low resistance of the patients is a risk factor..
D. The source of the infecting organism should be only exogenous.
E. Group A Streptococci is a common cause

199 **The most common types of nosocomial infections are**

A. Surgical wound and other soft tissue infections.
B. Urinary tract infections.
C. Respiratory infections.
D. Gastroenteritis.

E. Encephalitis.

200 **Factors most associated with an increased incidence of postoperative infections in the hospital are**

A. Over 60 years, of age.
B. Preoperative stay in hospital.
C. Long duration of the surgical procedure.
D. Pre-existing infection at the site of the wound.

E.   Patient with uncontroled hypertension.

201   The following are statements regarding surgical wound infections:

A.   Treatment with depilatories has been associated with a much higher frequency of infection.
B.   Staphylococcus aureus is the dominant species.
C.   They occurs commonly at the time of surgery.
D.   The main origin of the bacteria is from a member of the surgical team.
E.   Aerial transmission is a coomon mode of spread of infections.

202   The causal agents of infective endocarditis include

A.   *Streptococcus mutans.*
B.   *Pseudomonas aeruginosa.*
C.   *Haemophilus species.*
D.   *Escherichia coli.*

E.   *Bordetella pertussis.*

203   The following are statements regarding infective endocarditis:

A.   The sets blood culture are positive.
B.   Staphylococci are causative organisms.
C.   Janeway lesions are located on the palms or soles of the patient.
D.   patient is afebrile.

E.   cystoscopy is a predisposing factor.

204   Factors affect the control of hospital infections

A.   The lack of quality control of sterilization and disinfection procedures.
B.   The quality of water and food made available in the hospital.

C. The lack of trained staff.

D. The lack of knowledge of hospital infection control principles and practices among the staff.

E. The hospital environment itself.

205 **The following nosocomial pathogens are correctly matched with its infection**

A. *Staphylococcus epidermidis* :   i.v. infections.

B. *Escherichia coli*   :   urinary infections.

C. MRSA *S. aureus*   :   Bone infections.

D. *Pseudomonas* spp. :   GIT infection.

E. *Legionella* species   :   diarrhoea.

206 **The following are statements regarding roles of natural defense of the respiratory system:**

A. Epithelial layer of mucous memebrane secretes mucus which maintains moist surfaces and traps many microbes.

B. Cilia on mucous membranes of upper respiratory tract move upwards towards throat.

C. Nose hair filters dust, pollen, and microbes.

D. Coughing and sneezing expel foreign objects.

E. Lysozyme found in nasal secretions breaks down gram+ cell walls.

207 **The following are statements regarding pathogens of the respiratory system:**

A. Respiratory pathogens are easily transmitted from human to human.

B. All respiratory pathogens exist as part of the normal flora.

C. *Legionella* only infects the lung.

D. *Streptococcus* can cause infection in multiple sites of RT.

E. Most dangerous fungi are *Aspergillus* and *Pneumocystis*.

208 **The following bacteria is a common causative agent of following upper respiratory tract (URT)**

    A. *Haemophilus influenzae* : Laryngitis.
    B. *Streptococcus pneumoniae* : Epiglottitis.
    C. *Streptococcus pyogenes*. : Otitis media.
    D. *Streptococcus pyogenes* : sinusitis.

    E. *Streptococcus pyogenes* : Pharyngitis.

209 **The following are statements regarding pharyngitis:**

    A. Bacterial pharyngitis is more common than viral.
    B. Epstein–Barr virus is a causative of viral pharyngitis.
    C. Red pharyngeal mucosa is a presentation.
    D. Peak incidence of bacterial type is during the rainy season in the tropics.
    E. Viral pharyngitis is treated by antiviral drug.

210 **The following are statements regarding common cold:**

    A. It is a frequent occurrence, especially in young children.
    B. Its peak incidence during the winter period.
    C. The condition is caused mainly by *Streptococcus pyogenes*.
    D. Nasal discharge is a presentation.

    E. It is treated by antibiotics.

211 **Pneumocystis pneumonia**

    A. is caused by *Pneumocystis jirovecii*.
    B. causes life-threatening pneumonia amongimmunocompetent person.
    C. is common in patients with AIDS when the CD4 cell counts drop below 200/mm^3.
    D. causal agent has charateristics of both protozoan and fungus.

    E. treated with tetracycline.

212 The following are statements regarding influenza:

A. It is caused by influenza virus groups A–C.
B. Myalgia is common presentation.
C. Diagnosis is usually by laboratory investigation.
D
. *Staphylococcus aureus* can cause secondary bacterial pneumonia.
E. A vaccine is available, but it is only effective against newly isolated strains.

213 The following are statements regarding otitis media:

A. It is an inflammation of external auditory meatus.
B. Infection is most often caused by *S. pneumoniae* or *H. influenzae*.
C. It is most frequent in the younger child, whose Eustachian tube is shorter and more horizontal.
D
. Fever is a common feature.
E. Meningitis is a common complication. .

214 The following are statements regarding acute sinusitis:

A. It is most commonly caused by *S. pneumoniae* and *H. influenzae*.
B. There is impaired drainage of sinus secretions as a result of a prior upper respiratory tract infection or similar cause.
C. Headache is a presentation.
D
. Diagnosis is mainly by organism isolation.
E. Treatment is mainly by oral antibiotics.

215 The following are statements regarding laryngitis:

A. It is caused by one of the 'respiratory' viruses.
B. There is swelling and irritation of the voice box.
C. It is associated with hoarseness and loss of voice.

D. It may also be a feature of a common cold or influenza.

E. Specific antiviral therapy is required.

216 The following are statements regarding bronchitis:

A. Acute bronchitis is caused by *M. pneumonia.*
B. *H. influenzae* is cause of cute exacerbation of chronic bronchitis.
C. *S.pneumoniae* is a causative agent of Tracheobronchitis.
D. Sputum culture is of high diagnostic value.

E. Oral ampicillin is used in treatment.

217 The following are statements regarding scarlet fever:

A. It is caused by *Streptococcus pyogenes.*
B. It is usually seen in children under age of 18 years.
C. Symptoms usually begin with appearance of a rash.
D. Lymphadenopathy in neck is a finding.

E. It is treated by antibiotic therapies.

218 The following are statements regarding :

A. It is caused by the toxin produced by *Corynebacterium diphtheria.*
B. Can be accompanied by plaque-like pseudomembrane in the throat.
C. It is transmitted by direct contact with skin.
D. Effects of infection are due to the exotoxin.

E. It is difficult to treat it by antibiotics.

219 The following are statements regarding viral infections of the upper respiratory tract:

A. There are four types of single-stranded enveloped RNA

parainfluenza virus.
B. Transmission and pathology of parainfluenza virus similar to influenza virus.
C. Parainfluenza is a serious problem in adults.
D. Rhinoviruses are extremely small, non-enveloped, single-stranded RNA viruses.
E. Picornavirus infect nasopharynx because it has the same temperature for growth (33°C).

220 Bacterial infections of the lower respiratory tract include

A. Chlamydial pneumonia.
B. *Legionella* pneumonia.
C. Pertussis.
D. Inhalation anthrax.

E. Scarlet fever.

221 The following are statements regarding bacterial pneumonia:

A. It is characterized by inflammation of the alveoli and abnormal alveolar filling with fluid.
B. Cough is a typical symptom.
C. *Klebsiella pneumoniae* is one of causative agents.
D. Establishment of an infection in the lungs depends on the number of pathogens entering and the competence of the mucociliary escalator.
E. Bacterial pneumonia is treated with antibiotics.

222 The following pneumonias caused by different bacteria are correctly matched with clinical features:

A. *Streptococcus pneumoniae* : Sudden onset pleuritic pain, fever, rusty sputum, cold sores.
B. *Klebsiella pneumoniae* : Thick, viscous red sputum, alcoholic patient.
C. *Staphylococcus aureus* : Pneumonia following influenza.
D. *Streptococcus pneumoniae* : Pneumonia in the chronic bronchitic.

E.   *Mycoplasma pneumoniae* : Upper lobe consolidation, hilar lymphadenopathy, vagrant or alcoholic.

223   The following are statements regarding mycoplasma pneumonia:

A.   It is caused by *Mycoplasma pneumonia*.
B.   It is severe form of pneumonia.
C.   Accounts for about 10% of all pneumonias.
D.   Most common age for infections is between 20 and 40 years.
E.   Erythromycin is the drug of choice.

224   The following are statements regarding hospital-acquired pneumonia:

A.   It is the third most common nosocomial infection.
B.   Legionellas is the most common cause.
C.   Purulent sputum is a presentation.
D.   Bronchoalveolar lavage is the preferred method for collection of bacteriological specimens.
E.   Many patients respond well to optimal antimicrobial therapy.

225   Common bacterial causes of nosocomial pneumonia include

A.   *Staphylococcus aureus.*
B.   *Streptococcus pneumoniae.*
C.   *Pseudomonas aeruginosa.*
D.   *Mycobacterium tuberculosis.*
E.   *Klebsiella pneumonia.*

226   The following are statements regarding pulmonary tuberculosis:

A.   Chronic pneumonia is a common presentation of *M. tuberculosis.*
B.   It is common throughout the developing world.

C. Primary infection follows airborne transmission from an individual with pulmonary tuberculosis.

D. The thin cell wall of mycobacteria renders the organisms resistant to phagocytosis.

E. Primary tuberculous pneumonia only occurs if cell-mediated immunity is inadequate to resist the initial infective challenge.

227 The following are statements regarding diagnosis of pulmonary tuberculosis:

A. Clinically fever, night sweats, weight loss and haemoptysis are all should be clinical features.

B. The radiographic appearance supports one of the clinical presentations.

C. Routine Gram stain should be used.

D. Ziehl–Neelsen stain is acid fast stain.

E. The culture identification and susceptibility results take 48 hours.

228 The following are statements regarding pathogenesis of tuberculosis:

A. *M. tuberculosis* cell wall interferes with macrophage function.

B. *M. tuberculosis* cell wall inhibits the formation of the phagolysosome.

C. *M. tuberculosis* escape into the cytoplasm where it increases in number & eventually spreads to the lymph nodes.

D. Primary tuberculosis follows initial exposure to the pathogen.

E. Secondary tuberculosis occurs few weeks after the primary TB.

229 The following are statements regarding primary tuberculosis:

A. It occurs when a host encounters pathogen for the first time.

B. Organisms find their way to the alveoli when a localized

inflammatory response develops.
C.   Pathogens are coomonly killed in the alveoli.
D.   The type of immune response is mainly humoral immune response.
E.   Tubercles are aggregates of enlarged macrophages filled with bacteria.

230   **The following are statements regarding secondary tuberculosis:**

A.   It can be due to reactivation of old lesions.
B.   It could be due to gradual progression of primary tuberculosis into chronic disease.
C.   The incidence occur in majority of patients.
D.   It usually manifests itself in the apices of the lung.
E.   It usually occurs within two years of the primary infection.

231   **The following are statements regarding pertussis:**

A.   It is caused by *Bordetella pertussis*.
B.   The causative bacteria does not survive in the environment.
C.   Symptoms can be similar to those of a cold.
D.   Mortality is lowest in infants and children under 1 year old.
E.   Greatest numbers of infections are among 10-20 year-olds.

232   **The following are statements regarding empyema:**

A.   It is the accumulation of purulent fluid in the pleural space.
B.   Infection resulting from penetrating thoracic trauma is a route.
C.   Enterobacteriaceae is one of the causative agents.
D.   The collection of pus is required for diagnosis.
E.   It is treated by heavy antibotics.

233   **The following are statements regarding inhalation anthrax:**

A. The causative agent *Bacillus anthracis*.is *a g*ram-negative rod.
B. It produces a fulminate pneumonia comes on suddenly with great severity.
C. Antiphagocytic properties of the capsule aid its survival and growth in large numbers.
D. It leads to respiratory failure.
E. It is used recently as a biological weapon.

234   The following are statements regarding viral infections of the lower respiratory tract:

A. They cause majority of all acute respiratory tract infections.
B. Greatest incidence is among adults.
C. Influenza virus is a cause of majority of them.
D. Short incubation period of 1 to 4 days is a common characteristics of infection.
E. Direct transmission is through droplets.

235   The following are statements regarding fungal infections of the respiratory system:

A. *Pneumocystis (carinii) jiroveci is a cause of a lethal pneumonia common in AIDS patients.*
B. *Pneumocystis (carinii) jiroveci* is easily grown in culture.
C. Blastomycosis is increased in AIDS.
D. Fever, chills, and drenching sweats are presentation of blastomycosis.
E. Histoplasmosis affects people who live and work in the vicinity of bat or bird droppings.

236   The following are statements regarding aspergillosis:

A. Invasive aspergillosis shows a rapid progression to death.
B. Typically seen in the immunocompromised patients.
C. Fungus produces extracellular proteases, phospholipases, and toxic metabolites.

D. Seen more in nosocomial infections associated with air-conditioning systems.

E. Hemoptysis is absent in this infection.

237 **The following are statements regarding infections of gastrointestinal tract:**

A. Exogenous infections are brought in with contaminated food or water.

B. *C. difficile* and other exogenous infections are frequently acquired in hospital environments.

C. Exogenous infections can cause nausea and vomiting within 6 hours.

D. Endogenous infections are caused by organisms that are part of the normal flora.

E. *Streptococcus* is an example of exogenous infections.

238 **The following are statements regarding *Enterobacteriaceae*:**

A. O antigen is lipopolysaccharide in the outer membrane.

B. K antigen is surface polysaccharides.

C. H antigens are falgella proteins of motile strains.

D. Most of them colonize the upper gastrointestinal tract.

E. *Shigella* and *Salmonella* are part of the normal flora.

239 **The following are statements regarding enteric fever:**

A. It is a systemic infection focused in the gastrointestinal tract.

B. Abdominal pain is a prominent feature.

C. Diarrhea is severe from the 1st day of the infection.

D. Pathogenesis involves the penetration of enterocytes.

E. Pathogens spread to organs of the reticuloendothelial system.

240 **The following are statements regarding typhoid fever:**

A. It is caused by *Salmonella enterica* serotype Typhi..

B. The chronic carriers are the primary reservoir.
C. *S. Typhi* survive for short period inside viable host macrophages.
D. Systemic infection is exacerbated by release of lipopolysaccharide endotoxin.
E. The entire cycle takes only two weeks.

241 The following are statements regarding typhoid fever:

A. It is caused by invasive infection from small intestine into blood stream.
B. *Salmonella typhi* multiply in phagocytes resulting in septicemia.
C. Bacteria produce only exotoxin.
D. Transmitted by contaminated water or food.
E. Treated by broad spectrum antibiotic.

242 Toxin type of food poisoning can be caused by

A. *Salmonella Typhi.*
B. *Bacillus cereus.*
C. *Clostridium perfringens.*
D. *Staphylococcus aureus.*
E. *Streptococcus pyogenes.*

243 The following are statements regarding enteric fever:

AA. The stool culture is useful for the diagnosis during first week of illness.
BB. It is caused by *Salmonella Typhi* only.
CC. It can present with pea soup diarrhea.
DD. It is transmitted by the house flies.
E. Intestinal perforation is one of the complications.

244   The following are statements regarding typhoid fever:

A.   The temperature rises rapidly in the first week.
B.   Diarrhea can occur in the second week of onfection.
C.   Intestinal perforation in the distal ileum is a complication.
D.   It spread through poor hygiene habits.

E.   Widal test is a diagnostic.

245   The following are statements regarding salmonella gastroenteritis:

A.   It occurs in the intestine.
B.   It results from improper food handling.
C.   The chronic carriers are an important reservoir.
D.   *Salmonella enterica* can withstand the phagocytic response.

E.   Transcytosis and the inflammatory response cause the onset of diarrhea.

246   The following are statements regarding cholera:

A.   Cholera is an infection of the large intestine caused by the bacterium *Vibrio cholera.*
B.   Watery diarrhea is a main symptoms.
C.   Transmission occurs primarily by drinking water or eating contaminated food of an infected person.
D.   A rapid dip-stick test is to determine the presence of *V. cholera.*
E.   Oral rehydration therapy is the primary treatment.

247   The following are statements regarding cholera:

A.   It is caused by Gram negative curved rod.
B.   *V. cholerae* can grow in fresh or salt water.
C.   *V. cholerae* causes disease by release of exotoxin.
D.   Vaccine is inadequate to prevent the disease.

E.   Antibiotic therapy is the primary treatment.

248   The following are statements regarding Vibrio:

A.   It is highly motile by means of a single polar flagella.
B.   It can grow either aerobically or anaerobically.
C.   It has high tolerance for acidic conditions Grow well in
       mildly alkaline environments.
D.   Cell structure similar to that of Gram-negative bacteria.

E.   Its toxin causes a devastating intestinal infection.

249   The following are statements regarding Escherichia coli infection:

A.   Caused by Gram negative coliform.
B.   *Escherichia coli* commonly found as normal flora,
C.   Types of infection vary depending on the presence and type
       of exotoxins.
D.   Shiga-like toxins can result in mild diarrhea and nausea.

E.   Treatment by rehydration and controversial antibiotic
       treatment.

250   The following are statements regarding bacterial infections of GIT:

A.   *Streptococcus mutans* is one of the causes.
B.   *Helicobacter pylori* cause gastritis.
C.   *Clostridium difficile* causes antibiotic-associated
       enterocolitis.
D.   Toxins *of Clostridium difficile* produce pseudomembranes
       made up of fibrin and cells.
E.   Toxins produced by S.aureus causes slowly progressive
       gastroenteritis.

251   Most common bacterial foodborne pathogens are

A.   *Campylobacter jejuni.*

B. *Clostridium perfringens.*
C. *Salmonella* spp.
D. *Escherichia coli.*

E. *Brucella* spp.

252   The following are statements regarding food poisoning:

A. It appear suddenly and within 48 hours after ingestion of food contaminated with a pathogen.
B. Abdominal cramping is symptom.
C. Infective agents include viruses, bacteria, and parasites.
D. Food poisoning caused by Salmonella bacteria gives victims flu-like symptoms for as long as 48 hours.
E. Staphylococcal food poisoning appears about 48 hours after eating contaminated food.

253   Symptoms of food poisoning include

A. abdominal cramps.
B. diarrhea (may be bloody).
C. fever and chills.
D. severe abdominal pain.

E. nausea and vomiting.

254   The following are statements regarding food poisoning:

A. *Staphylococcus aureus* enterotoxin is a superantigen.
B. Diarrhea caused by *Staphylococcus aureus* is a typical feature of this kind of food poisoning.
C. *B. cereus* is associated with reheated fried rice.
D. Ingestion of *B. cereus* exotoxin produces mild symptoms.

E. Shiga toxin causes inflammation and bleeding.

255   The following are statements regarding food poisoning:

A. Infectious agents include viruses, bacteria, and parasites.
B. Toxic agents include fungal toxins (poisonous mushrooms).

C. Low -level contamination with salmonella may result in a food poisoning-like syndrome.
D. Mortality of Salmonella spp due to septic shock caused by endotoxin.
E. *Campylobacter jejuni* usually transmitted in cow's milk and related products.

256   The following are statements regarding *Helicobacter pylori*:

A. They are similar to *Campylobacter* in morphology and growth characteristics.
B. Lipopolysaccharides in the outer layer is less toxic than those in other Gram-negative pathogens.
C. Production of a urease Allows it to survive in very acidic environments.
D. It produces a vacuolating cytotoxin.

E. Infected cells have large vacuoles throughout their cytoplasm.

257   The following are statements regarding peptic ulcer caused by *Helicobacter pylori*:

A. *Helicobacter pylori* has multiple polar knobbed flagella.
B. Urease is a virulence factor of bacteria.
C. Weight gain is a presentation.
D. Diagnosed by assessing damage to stomach lining and isolation of urease+, Gram- vibrios.
E. Perforations of stomach or intestine is a complication.

258   The following are statements regarding watery diarrhea:

A. It is caused by enterotoxin-secreting bacteria.
B. Enterotoxigenic *Escherichia coli is cause.*
C. Watery diarrhea caused by *V. cholerae* uasually resolve in 3 to 7 days.
D. May be accompanying by vomiting and fever.

E.   Usually self-limiting.

259   The following are statements regarding traveler's diarrhea:

A.   Enterotoxigenic strains of *E. coli.* Is acause.
B.   Majority are caused by *Shigella..*
C.   Usually brief and self-limiting.
D   The major source is ingestion of improperly cooked food.

E.   Typically involves multiple patients.

260   The following are statements regarding nosocomial gastrointestinal infections:

A.   E. coli is one of a major causative pathogen.
B.   Contaminated food prepared outside the hospital is a source.
C.   *C. difficile* accounts for 90% of infections.
D   Symptoms are usually only mild diarrhea.

E.   Colitis arises either during or after treatment with antibiotics.

261   The following are statements regarding shigella:

A.   Shigella is like E.coli both can ferment lactose.
B.   *S. dysenteriae* produces most of Shiga toxin.
C.   Shigellosis is one of the most common causes of diarrhea worldwide.
D   *S. dysenteriae* causes bacillary dysentery.

E.   There is direct connection between *Shigella* infections and community sanitary practices.

262   The following are statements regarding pathogenesis of shigellosis:

A.   *Shigella* is affected by human gastric acid.
B.   *Shigella* causes mucosal ulcerations and abscess formation.

C.	There is cell-to-cell extensions cause localized ulcers in the mucosa, particularly in colon.
D.	*Shigella* lyses the vacuole membranes.
E.	Shiga toxin causes less severity of the illness.

**263	The following are statements regarding Campylobacter enteritis:**

A.	It is caused by *Campylobacter jejuni*.
B.	The primary reservoir is human.
C.	Undercooked poultry is the most common source.
D.	Bacteria adhere to and enter cells in endocytic vacuoles.

E.	Illness begins about 2 weeks after ingestion includes fever and lower abdominal pain.

**264	The following are statements regarding viral infections of the digestive system:**

A.	Diarrhea is the most common sign of infection.
B.	Diarrhea lasts for at least 30 days.
C.	There is abundant excretion of virions in the stool.
D.	Virus must be detected in ill patients.

E.	Must be has a significant antibody response.

**265	Specific criteria must be met to implicate viruses in digestive infections include:**

A.	Virus must be detected in non-ill and ill patients.
B.	Viral shedding must correlate with onset of symptoms.
C.	Disease must be reproduced by experimental inoculation of non-immune humans or animals.
D.	Must be a significant antibody response.

E.	Other causes of the signs and symptoms must be excluded.

**266	Viruses that can cause gastrointestinal infections are**

A. Rotavirus.
B. Calicivirus.
C. Astrovirus.
D. Some serotypes of adenovirus.
E. Enterovirus.

267   The following are statements regarding Rotavirus:

A. It is enveloped spherical virus.
B. It has a double-capsid structure.
C. It is a cause of less than 10% of cases of acute gastroenteritis.
D. Outbreaks of rotavirus infections common in adults.
E. Malabsorption is the end result of infection.

268   The following are statements regarding Enterovirus:

A. Enteroviruses are members of the *picornaviridae.*
B. They can survive in the stomach.
C. Humans are the natural hosts.
D. Symptomatic infection is common.
E. Virus will normally spend 1 to 4 weeks in the oropharynx.

269   The following are statements regarding Hepatitis A:

A. It is classified as a member of the genus *hepatovirus,* family *picornaviridae.*
B. It is non-enveloped, double-stranded RNA virus.
C. They have many serotype.
D. Transmission is usually via the fecal-oral route.
E. Seen in feces 10-14 days before onset of symptom.

270   The following are statements regarding Hepatitis A:

A. Virus replicates initially in intestinal mucosa.
B. It causes necrosis of the parenchymal cells.
C. Patients with antibodies can be reinfected.
D. Incubation times vary from 10 to 50 days,
E. Stool can become clay-colored 1 to 5 days before onset of jaundice.

271 The following are statements regarding Hepatitis B:

A. It is classified as a member of family *picornaviridae*.
B. It is a DNA virus.
C. It has spherical shape with a surrounding envelope.
D. Its envelope contains viral surface antigens HBsAg.
E. It is used as a template for reverse transcription.

272 The following are statements regarding Hepatitis B infection:

A. Majority of those infected become chronic carriers.
B. 50% of infections are sexually transmitted.
C. Tattooing or piercing can easily transmit this viral infection.
D. Lesions in acute hepatitis B infections resemble those seen with other hepatitis viruses.
E. Screening of blood donors has markedly reduced the incidence of transfusion transmission.

273 The following are statements regarding Hepatitis B infection:

A. Incubation time is 7-160 days.
B. Loss of appetite is a presentation of acute infection.
C. Chronic active infection causes a continued inflammation resulting in necrosis of hepatocytes.
D. Progressive fibrosis is a finding.
E. Majority of infected individuals will develop chronic hepatitis.

274   The following are statements regarding Hepatitis C:

A.   Classified as a member of the *flaviviridae* family.
B.   It is DNA virus.
C.   It has six major genotypes and multiple subtypes.
D.   It transmitted by blood transfusions.
E.   Hemodialysis patients are also at risk.

275   The following are statements regarding Hepatitis C:

A.   Incubation time is 4-6 weeks.
B.   Infection is usually severe.
C.   Majority of those infected will become carriers of the infection.
D.   Hepato cellular carcinoma is a late consequences of chronic hepatitis C infection.
E.   Hepatitis C is the leading cause of liver transplants.

276   The following are statements regarding Hepatitis D:

A.   It is double-stranded DNA virus.
B.   It requires the presence of hepatitis C.
C.   Seen most often in intravenous drug abusers.
D.   Recurrence of jaundice occurs in superinfection with hepatitis D.
E.   Interferon-α is given to doubly infected patients.

277   The following are statements regarding Hepatitis E:

A.   It is classified in the family *caliciviridae*.
B.   It is non-enveloped DNA virus.
C.   It is transmitted by the fecal-oral route.
D.   Infection is frequently subclinical.
E.   The incubation time is about 40 days.

278   The following are statements regarding Hepatitis G:

A. Classified in the family *flaviviridae*.
B. It is similar to hepatitis B.
C. RNA virus.
D 2% of blood donors are positive for hepatitis G RNA.
.
E. No treatment is available.

279 The infection which associated with the strain of *Escherichia coli* include:

A. Neonatal meningitis.
B. Urinary tract infection.
C. Haemolytic uraemic syndrome.
D Bacillary dysentery.
.
E. Enteric Fever.

280 The following bacteria that biochemically ferment with lactose sugar include

A *Esherichia coli.*
B. *Salmonella typhi.*
C. *Shigella boydii.*
D *Klebsiella pneumonia.*
E. *Pseudomonas aeruginosa.*

281 Following infections can be transmitted from mother to fetus via placenta.

A. Typhoid.
B. Malaria.
C. Syphilis.
D. AIDS.
E. Rubella.

282 Common uropathogens include

A. *Escherichia coli.*
B. *Proteus.*
C. *Pseudomonas aeruginosa.*
D. *Mycobacterium tuberculosis.*
E. *Staphylococcus aureus.*

283   Commensal microflora of the urethra include

A. *Staphylococci saprophyticus.*
B. *Viridans and non-hemolytic streptococci.*
C. *Lactobacilli.*
D. *Corynebacterium urealyticum.*
E. *Saprophytic Neisseria.*

284   Common risk factors for urinary tract infection in women

A. Urinary tract obstruction.
B. Hypertension.
C. Pregnancy.
D. Sexual intercourse.
E. Estrogen deficiency.

285   Common risk factors for urinary tract infection in men include

A. Urinary tract obstruction.
B. Prostatic enlargement.
C. Urologic instrumentation or surgery.
D. Hydrocele.
E. Lack of circumcision.

286   The following are statements regarding UTI:

A. Hematogenous route of infection is the most common.
B. Colonization of urethra and periurethral tissue by uropathogens the initial event.
C. Hospital infection associated with lower urinary tract

instrumentation.

D. Enteric bacteria is source of uropathogens.

E. Papillary necrosis: complication of pyelonephritis.

287 The following are statements regarding bacterial virulence factors in UTI:

A. *Escherichia coli* strains expressing O-antigens cause high proportion of infections.
B. Gram-negative endotoxin decreases ureteral peristalsis.
C. K6 antigens of *E. coli* associated with antiphagocytic activity.
D. P-fimbriated *E. coli* is a cause of pyelonephritis.

E. *Hemolysin* produced by many uropathogens damages renal tubular epithelium and promotes invasive infection.

288 The following are statements regarding host protective factors in UTI:

A. Flushing mechanism of micturition.
B. Low vaginal pH (3.5-4.5) suppresses colonization by uropathogens.
C. Normal acid pH of urine (4.6-6) is anti-bacterial
D. Urinary Tamm-Horsefall protein blocks *Staph aureas* attachment to uroepithelial cells.
E. Chemotactic interleukin-8 eradicate bacteriuria

289 The following are statements regarding signs and symptoms of UTI:

A. Fever is high in lower UTI.
B. Frequent and painful urination in lower UTI.
C. Occasional suprapubic pain or sensation of heaviness in lower UTI.
D. Flank pain is present in upper UTI.
E. Fever and chills in upper UTI.

290   Indications for urinalysis and culture

A.   Symptoms suggestive of infection like dysuria.
B.   Suspicion of complicated infection as fever.
C.   Atypical symptoms.
D.   Failure to respond to initial therapy.
E.   Recurrent symptoms < 2 weeks after treatment for a previous UTI not cultured.

291   Factors affecting growth & colony count of bacteria in urine

A.   Urine pH.
B.   Urine constituents.
C.   Urine flow rate.
D.   Residual urine volume.
E.   Urinary antiseptics.

292   Anaerobic infections

A.   can be associated with gas in tissues.
B.   are usually present with foul-smelling discharge.
C.   are rarely associated with contamination of normal flora.
D.   are sometimes polymicrobial nature.
E.   cannot be treated with antimicrobial drugs.

293   The following microorganism can cause urinary tract infection.

A.   *Candida albicans.*
B.   *Streptococcocus agalactiae.*
C.   *Salmonella Typhi.*
D   *Escherichia coli.*
.
E.   *Staphylococcus saprophyticus.*

294   The following are statements regarding non-gonoccocal urethritis (NGU) :

A. Chlamydia trachomatis accounts for a majority of NGU.
B. One of the implicated organism in NGU is *Haemophilus influenzae*.
C. *Rickettsia prowazekii* infection leads to severe form of NGU.
D. Serology (ELISA/Latex agglutination test) is the mainstay for diagnosing NGU.
E. The majority of NGU cases are asymptomatic.

295 Microorganisms which can be used as potential biological weapon include

A. *Brucella abortus.*
B. *Leptospira interrogans.*
C. *Yersinia pestis.*
D. *Bacillus anthracis.*

E. *Mycobacteria leprae.*

296 The following are statements regarding diagnostic tests of UTI:

A. Bacterial count >100,000 /ml indicative of infection in urinanalysis.
B. Nitrite dipstick test the presence of protein.
C. Leukocyte esterase test identifies WBC in urine.
D. Gram stain of urine is obtained by clean catch urine.

E. Urine culture and sensitivity identify infecting organism and most effective antibiotic.

297 The following are statements regarding diagnostic tests for adults who have recurrent infections or persistent bacteriuria:

A. Intravenous pyelography (IVP) evaluates structure and excretory function of kidneys, ureters, and bladder.
B. Barium enema is used to visualize the internal structures.
C. Voiding cystourethrography is to assess bladder and urethra

when filled and during voiding.

D. Cystoscopy is used for diagnostic, tissue biopsy, interventions.

E. Manual pelvic or prostate examinations to assess structural changes of genitourinary tract.

298 **The following are statements regarding possible outcomes of treatment for UTI, determined by follow-up urinalysis and culture:**

A. Cure; no pathogens in urine.
B. Unresolved bacteriuria.
C. Persistent bacteriuria or relapse.
D. Development of new infection with different pathogen.
E. No pathogen bacteria with a lot of WBS.

299 **The following are statements regarding urethritis:**

A. It is often associated with sexually transmitted pathogens.
B. Frequency is presentation.
C. Painless urination is a presentation.
D. Urine is cloudy.
E. Treatment start when microorganism counts is 100,000/ml.

300 **The following are statements regarding acute cystitis:**

A. It is caused mainly by E. coli.
B. Painless urination is a presentation.
C. The incidence among men more than women.
D. Urine is cloudy and malodorous.
E. Leukocyte esterase positive.

301 **The following are statements regarding acute pyelonephritis:**

A. Blood stream is a route of invasion.

B.   Both kidneys are always affected.
C.   Fever and chills are common presentations.
D.   Leukocytosis is present.

E.   It require IV antibiotics.

302   The following are statements regarding chronic pyelonephritis:

A.   It is a chronic tubulointerstitial inflammation involving renal parenchyma.
B.   Leads to scarring of pelvis and calyces.
C.   Chronic inflammatory infiltrates.
D.   Decrease incidence of preterm labor in pregnancy.

E.   Papillary necrosis is a complication.

303   The following are statements regarding catheter-associated UTI:

A.   Long term catheter bacteriuria is inevitable.
B.   40% of nosocomial infections.
C.   Most common source of gram-positive bacteremia.
D.   Asymptomatic bacteriuria should not treated unless they are immunosuppressed.
E.   Severe infection needs IV antibiotics.

304   The following are statements regarding pregnancy and urinary tract infections:

A.   There is increased risk of kidney infections in pregnancy.
B.   During pregnancy, high progesterone levels elevate the risk of symptomatic bacteriuria.
C.   If bacteriuria is present they do have a high risk of a kidney infection.
D.   A kidney infection during pregnancy may result in premature birth or pre-eclampsia.
E.   Treatment is recommended when urine testing shows signs of an infection even in the absence of symptoms.

305   **The following are statements regarding fungal urinary tract infections:**

A.   Candida albicans is the most common cause.
B.   Diabetes is a predisposing factors
C.   Ascending infection is common
D.   Urine urine leukocytosis is a finding.
E.   Urine fungal culture catheterization for fungal culture is used in diagnosis.

306   **Nosocomial pathogens include**

A.   *Clostridium difficile.*
B.   *Staphylococcus aureus.*
C.   *Clostridium tetani.*
D.   *Helicobacter pylori.*
E.   *Pseudomonas aeruginosa.*

307   **The following are statements regarding vaginitis and vaginosis:**

A.   Symptoms depend on the etiologic agent.
B.   *Candida albicans* is initially normal biota living in low numbers.
C.   White vaginal discharge occurs in *Candida albicans* infection.
D.   Vaginal discharge with a very fishy odor, especially after sex is characteristic of ifection by *Gardnerella* species.
E.   Itching is uncommon in *Gardnerella* species.

308   **The following are statements regarding gonorrhea:**

A.   *N. gonorrhoeae* is the etiologic agent.
B.   It is commonly spread from the urethra to epididymis in male patients.

C. It leads to infertility in majority of infected men.
D. Mucopurulent or bloody vaginal discharge is a presentation in women.
E. Pelvic inflammatory disease is a compication in women.

309 The following are statements regarding gonorrhea:

A. It is caused by bacteria *Neisseria gonorrhea*.
B. It is leading cause of sterility in men.
C. Endocarditis is a complication.
D. It is diagnosed by a smear of the discharge.

E. It is treated with antibiotics.

310 The following are statements regarding gonorrhea:

A. Majority of women asymptomatic carriers.
B. May cause Pelvic Inflammatory Disease (PID) in women.
C. Man develops a drip, pus exudate 3-8 days after exposure
D. Painful urination in women

E. If newborn has contact with the bacteria during birth may cause blindness

311 Specific serological tests for syphilis are

A. VDRL test
B. FTA-ABS test.
C. EIA.
D. TPI test.
E. Rapid plasma reagin test.

312 The following are statements regarding Chlamydia:

A. Majority of cases are symptomatic.
B. Symptoms mimicking gonorrhea in male patients.
C. Cervicitis is a presentation in women.
D. All strains can invade the lymphatic tissues resulting in

.   lymphogranuloma venereum.
E. Babies born to mothers with infections can develop eye infections and pneumonia.

313 The following are statements regarding classification of sexually-transmitted diseases:

A. *Gonorrhea* is a mucosal infection.
B. Papillomavirus is a systemic infections.
C. HIV is a systemic infections.
D. Herpes simplex is ulcerative infections.
E. Chancroid is ulcerative infections.

314 Factors that affect the transmission of STDs

A. Age.
B. Gender.
C. Genetic susceptibility.
D. Smoking.
E. Circumcision in males.

315 The following are statements regarding chlamydial infection:

A. It affects young adults more than teenagers.
B. It may have been acquired in the remote past.
C. Around 5% of infected sexual partners in males.
D. ~ 50% of infected sexual partners in women.
E. Urethritis occurs in both males and females.

316 The following are statements regarding microbiology of gonorrhea:

A. It is strict human pathogen.
B. It is Gram-positive diplococcus
C. IgA protease (cleaves IgA).

D   Oxidase-positive.
.

E.   Fastidious growth.

317   Virulence determinants of Neisseria gonorrhoeae include

A.   pilus colonization factor.
B.   opa proteins.
C.   Lipooligosaccharide.
D   IgA1 protease.
.

E.   Transferrin.

318   The following are statements regarding *Chlamydia trachomatis*:

A.   It is obligate intracellular bacteria.
B.   It is Gram negative bacteria.
C.   It has 2-stage life cycle.
D   Reticulated body is vegetative like.
.

E.   Treatmented by tetracyclines .

319   The following are statements regarding syphilis causative bacteria:

A.   *Treponema pallidum* is a spirochete and labile spiral bacterium.
B.   Man and animal are recognized hosts.
C.   It is non-cultivable bacteria.
D.   It is Gram-negative like.
E.   It has axial filaments.

320   The following are statements regarding microbiology of chancroid:

A.   It is caused by *Haemophilus ducreyi*.
B.   Gram-positive coccobacilli.

C. Fastidious and labile.
D. Diagnosis is usually clinical, by exclusion of other agents of genital ulcers.
E. Females >> Males.

321 The following are statements regarding pelvic inflammatory disease:

A. It is caused by gonorrhea only.
B. It is an infection of the fallopian tubes, uterus and ovaries.
C. It causes sterility in women.
D. There is scarring of fallopian tubes lead to ectopic pregnancies.
E. Treated with antibiotics.

322 The following are statements regarding genital warts:

A. HPV types 6 and 11 are most frequently the cause of genital warts.
B. It increased the risk for endometrial cancer.
C. Warts on genitalia 2 weeks to 8 months after exposure.
D. It is spread through direct skin-to-skin contact.
E. Genital warts are commonly occur singly.

323 The following are statements regarding Herpes genitalis:

A. Refers to a genital infection by Herpes simplex virus.
B. Most individuals carrying herpes are unaware about the infection.
C. Genital HSV-2 infections are the cause of majority of infections.
D. Herpes is asymptomatic in the majority of cases.
E. In males, the lesions occur on the glans penis.

324 The following are statements regarding genital Herpes in women:

A. Increase chance of miscarriages.
B. Increase cervical cancer risk.
C. The treatment eradicates the symptome and viruses.
D   Stress leads to reoccurs at times.
.
E. Acyclovir is the drug of choice.

325 The following are statements regarding human papillomavirus (HPV):

A. It is an RNA virus from the papillomavirus family.
B. Majority of the known types of HPV cause symptoms in most people.
C. Most HPV infections in young women are temporary and have little long-term significance.
D   There is high risk of developing precancerous lesions of the
.   cervix.
E. High-risk sexually transmitted HPVs lead to the development of cervical intraepithelial neoplasia (CIN).

4.1 Questions with answers: (True/False questions):

141 The following age group is correctly matched with the most common causative microorganism of osteomyelitis:

T   A. Newborns (younger than 4) : group A and B *Streptococcus* species.

T   B. Children (aged 4 to 4 y) : *S. aureus*, group A *Streptococcus* species.

T   C. Children, adolescents (aged 4 y to adult) : *S. aureus* .

F   D Adult   : *Streptococcus* species.
.

T   E. Sickle cell anemia patients : *Salmonella* species .

142   The following are statements regarding osteomyelitis (OM):

T   A. It can be subclassified on the basis of the causative organism.

T   B. Chronic OM is often defined as OM that has been present for more than one month.

T   C. Microorganisms may infect bone via the bloodstream.

T   D Pus spreads into the bone's blood vessels, impairing their
.   flow, and areas of devitalized infected bone, known as *sequestra*,

F   E. Involucrum is the area of necrosis.

143   The following are statements regarding osteomyelitis:

T   A. In children, the long bones are usually affected.

T   B. In adults, the vertebrae and the pelvis are most commonly affected.

T   C. Acute osteomyelitis almost invariably occurs in children.

F   D Osteomyelitis is a secondary complication in majority of
.   patients with pulmonary tuberculosis.

T   E. In tubercular osteomyelitis, the long bones and vertebrae are the ones that tend to be affected.

144   The following are statements regarding osteomyelitis:

T   A. *Staphylococcus aureus* is the organism most commonly isolated from all forms of osteomyelitis.

F   B. Bloodstream-sourced osteomyelitis is seen most frequently in adults.

T   C. *Blastomyces dermatitidis* is the two most common cause of mycotic osteomyelitis.

T D. Diagnosis of osteomyelitis is often based on radiologic results showing a lytic center with a ring of sclerosis.

T E. Presence of sepsis is commonly complicate osteomyelitis.

145 The following are statements regarding Brodie abscess:

T A. It is a subacute osteomyelitis, which may persist for years before converting to a frank osteomyelitis.

T B. It is a well-defined cavity in cancellous bone

T C. Nocturnal localized pain is a clinical presentation.

F D. Brodie's abscess is best visualized using X-ray.

F E. The treatment of choice is by antibiotics.

146 The following are statements regarding acute septic arthritis:

T A. Direct invasion is the route of Infection.

T B. Haemophilus influenzae is a causative organism.

T C. Acute synovitis with purulent joint effusion is a finding.

T D. Blood culture is used in investigation.

T E. Complete recovery is a sequelae.

147 The following are statements regarding tuberculosis of bone and joint:

T A. It is particularly likely to attack the spine and the ends of the long bones.

T B. If not treated, the spinal segments may collapse and cause paralysis in one or both legs.

T C. Tuberculous granuloma is a finding.

T D. Present with abscess or kyphosis.

F E. Joint aspiration for AAFB identified in majority of patients.

148 The following are statements regarding Viral exanthems:

F   A.   They are more common among adults.

T   B.   In children, they are most often related to infection.

T   C.   Determining the cause of an exanthem is based on the characteristic morphology, distribution and time course of the eruption.

T   D.   Measles is caused by a ssRNA virus belonging to the *Paramyxoviridae* family.

T   E.   The measles's eruption typically resolves in the same order as its appearance.

149   The following are statements regarding Measles:

T   A.   It has an incubation period of approximately 10–12 days.

T   B.   Koplik spots is seen during the prodromal phase.

F   C.   Typical exanthem begins from the 1st day of infection.

T   D.   Transient immunosuppression is a complications.

F   E.   It is treated by antiviral therapy.

150   The following are statements regarding Rubella:

T   A.   It is caused by an RNA virus in the *Togaviridae* family.

F   B.   Majority of infected individuals become symptomatic.

T   C.   A maculopapular exanthem appears after approximately 2–5 days.

T   D.   The diagnosis of rubella can be made with IgM antibody titers.

T   E.   Congenital rubella syndrome is the most serious complication.

151   The following are statements regarding erythema infectiosum:

T   A.   It is a common childhood exanthematous illness caused by parvovirus B19.

F   B.   Patients present with fiery-red facial erythema after incubation period for 3-4 weeks.

T   C.   The exanthem recurs intermittently in response to stimuli, such as local irritation, high temperatures and emotional stress.

T   D.   An ELISA is commercially available with high sensitivity in

.   diagnosis.
T   E.   PCR can detect viral DNA in patient's urine.

152   The following are statements regarding Roseola Infantum:

T   A.   It is caused by human herpesvirus types 6 and 7.
F   B.   By the end of the second year of life, approximately half of all children are seropositive for HHV-6.
T   C.   The incubation period is 5–15 day.
T   D   Roseola infection can cause leukopenia.
.
F   E.   The diagnosis of roseola is made by laboratory detection of HHV-6 and -7.

153   The following are statements regarding Epstein–Barr Virus infection:

T   A.   Epstein–Barr virus (EBV) is a member of the *Herpesvirus* family, belonging to the genus *Lymphocryptovirus.*
F   B.   Half of children infected with EBV manifest an exanthema.
T   C.   A characteristic bright-red morbilliform eruption almost always occurs if mpicillin is administered to the infected child.
T   D   The eruption most likely results from ampicillin–antibody
.   immune complexes as a consequence of polyclonal B-cell activation.
F   E.   This reaction is considered a true drug allergy.

154   The following are statements regarding Varicella & Herpes Zoster:

F   A.   Varicella is caused by varicella-zoster virus (VZV), an enveloped RNA virus.
F   B.   The transmission of virus requires skin-to-skin contact.
T   C.   The virus initially undergoes primary replication, beginning 3–4 days after exposure.
T   D   The exanthem begins soon after as erythematous pruritic
.   macules.
T   E.   Bacterial superinfection is the most common complication of

varicella.

155   The following are statements regarding Eczema Herpeticum:

T   A.   It is a severe form of disseminated cutaneous HSV infection, which occurs primarily in individuals with atopic dermatitis.

T   B.   Defective cytokine secretion in skin appear to play a role in the pathogenesis.

T   C.   Patients present with monomorphic umbilicated vesiclulopustules.

T   D.   The diagnosis is made clinically.

F   E.   Topical steroids is the drug of choice.

156   The following are statements regarding Hand–Foot–Mouth Disease:

T   A.   It is an exanthem caused by viruses of the *Picornaviridae* family in the *Enterovirus* genus.

T   B.   The most common pathogen is the Coxsackie A16 virus.

F   C.   The infection has a typical incubation period of 10-15 days.

F   D.   Appearance of painful oval, gray vesicles is the main manifestation followed by fever and lymphadenopathy.

T   E.   The vesicles are often arranged parallel to the dermatoglyphs.

157   The following are statements regarding papular acrodermatitis of childhood (PAC):

T   A.   It is a unique cutaneous disorder characterized by the abrupt onset of an erythematous papular exanthema.

F   B.   It is primarily affecting children between 8 and 12 years of age.

F   C.   it was believed that PAC is a manifestation of hepatitis A infection.

T   D.   Occasionally, the papules coalesce into larger plaques and become hemorrhagic or form scales.

F   E.   Treatment is by antiviral therapy.

158   The following are statements regarding papular purpuric glove and socks syndrome (PPGSS):

T   A.   It is usually caused by parovovirus B19.
T   B.   Clinically, it is characterized by symmetric, painful erythema, and edema of the hands and feet that later progresses to a petechial rash.
F   C.   Edema and erythema cann't be observed on the buccal and genital mucosa.
T   D.   Patients with PPGSS are contagious when they exhibit the exanthem.
T   E.   Treatment is symptomatic.

159   The following are statements regarding Impetigo:

T   A.   It is always caused by b-hemolytic streptococci and/or *S. aureus*.
F   B.   Its peak incidence is among children aged 10-12 years.
T   C.   It is usually occurs on exposed areas of the body, most frequently the face and extremities.
T   D.   During the course of 2– 3 weeks, streptococcal strains transferred from the skin lesions to the upper respiratory tract.
F   E.   The anti–streptolysin O response is strong in patients with streptococcal impetigo.

160   The following are statements regarding cutaneous abscesses:

F   A.   *S. aureus* is usually the causative pathogen in majority of cases.
F   B.   The inflammation and purulence occur as infectious complication.
T   C.   High fever is a presentation.
F   D.   Gram stain and culture are commonly uased in diagnosis.
T   E.   Extensive surrounding cellulitis, is a complication.

161   The following are statements regarding furuncles:

T   A.   They are usually caused by *S. aureus*.

T B. They differ from folliculitis, in which inflammation is more superficial and pus is present in the epidermis.

F C. They occur mainly in hairy scalp.

T D. The lesion consists of an inflammatory nodule and an overlying pustule through which hair emerges.

F E. Systemic antibiotics are usually necessary in treatment.

162 The following are statements regarding erysipelas:

F A. It affects the deeper dermis, as well as subcutaneous fat.

F B. It is more common among adults between 20-40 years.

T C. It is almost always caused by b-hemolytic streptococci (usually group A).

T D. Penicillin is the treatment of choice.

T E. The prognosis is excellent.

163 The following are statements regarding cellulitis:

T A. It is an acute spreading infection of the skin, extending more deeply than erysipelas to involve the subcutaneous tissues.

F B. It is almost always caused by b-hemolytic streptococci (usually group A).

T C. Rapidly spreading areas of edema is a manifestation.

F D. Systemic manifestations are usually severe.

T E. Blood culture results are positive in majority of cases.

164 The following are statements regarding necrotizing skin and soft-tissue infections:

T A. They are often deep and devastating.

T B. They are usually secondary infections.

F C. They are usually monomicrobial (streptococci).

T D. Presence of gas in the soft tissues is a clinical feature.

T E. They require operative intervention.

165 The following are statements regarding necrotizing fasciitis:

T   A.   Insect bite is an initial lesion.
T   B.   *S. pyogenes* is causative microorganism.
F   C.   Approximately two-third of cases in the upper extremities.
T   D   Diabetes is an underlying cause.
.

T   E.   In the polymicrobial form, an average of 5 pathogens different anaerobic and aerobic organisms can be cultured from the involved fascial plane in each wound.

166   The following are statements regarding anaerobic streptococcal myositis:

F   A.   It causes a less indolent infection than other streptococci.
T   B.   It is usually associated with trauma or a surgical procedure.
T   C.   Incision and drainage are critical.
T   D   Antibiotic treatment is highly effective.
.

T   E.   Penicillin or ampicillin should be administered in high doses.

167   The following are statements regarding pyomyositis:

T   A.   It is caused mainly by *S. aureus*.
F   B.   Blood culture results are positive in majority of cases.
T   C.   Localized pain in a single muscle group is a presenting finding.
F   D   The disease occurs most often in trunk muscles.
.

T   E.   Antibiotics plus extensive surgical incision and drainage are required for appropriate management.

168   The following are statements regarding fournier gangrene:

T   A.   It involves the scrotum and penis or vulva.
F   B.   The mean age of onset is 30 years.
F   C.   Most cases are caused by *S. aureus*.
T   D.   Most patients initially have a urinary tract tract.
T   E.   Aggressive surgical exploration and appropriate

debridement is necessary to remove all necrotic tissue.

169   The following are statements regarding clostridial myonecrosis:

F   A.   *C. novyi* is the most frequent cause of trauma associated gas gangrene.
T   B.   *C. septicum* is the causative of spontaneous gangrene.
T   C.   Skin may initially be pale.
T   D.   Gas in the tissue, detected as crepitus.
F   E.   Tetracycline is the drug of choice.

170   The following are statements regarding anthrax:

F   A.   The incubation period of 14-20 days.
T   B.   Regional lymphadenopathy is common presentation.
T   C.   Blood culture results are almost always negative.
T   D.   Immunohistochemical staining is useful in duagnosis
T   E.   Penicillin is effective therapy.

171   The following are statements regarding malasseziosis:

T   A.   There are Hypo- to hyperpigmented patches with scales.
T   B.   Can cause folliculitis.
T   C.   These fungi also cause dandruff.
T   D.   Presence of sphaghetti and meatballs of oval to round budding yeasts is diagnostic.
F   E.   It is treated by excessive washing by soap.

172   The following are statements regarding dermatophytoses:

T   A.   *Microsporum* is a cause.
T   B.   It may acquired from other animals.
T   C.   Microscopic observation of fungal elements in skin samples is diagnostic.
T   D.   Human genetics may play a role in making some families more susceptible to some of these fungi.
F   E.   Corporis type is treated by systemically applied doses of

fluconazole.

173 The following are statements regarding pityriasis versicolor:

T A. Malassezia furfur is an etiological agent.
T B. An asymtomatic benign infection of the stratum corneum layer of skin.
F C. It is common in cold climate.
F D. Diagnosis commonly require for tissue biopsies.
T E. The confirmatory test is by direct microscopy of skin scrapings mounted in 10% potassium hydroxide.

174 The following are statements regarding Eumycetoma:

T A. It is a chronic subcutaneous infection that can spread to bone and lymph tissue.
T B. Formation of grains (colonies) is characteristic.
T C. It is caused by Aerobic actinomycetes.
T D. The disease develops typically as a result of a minor trauma that implants the etiological agent.
F E. It is self-limited disease.

175 The following are statements regarding chromoblastomycosis:

T A. It is a chronic skin fungal infection.
F B. Fungal agents are whitely pigmented.
T C. Lesions are nodular and verrucous.
T D. Infections tend to be of the lower extremities.
T E. *Fonsecea pedrosoi* is causative agent.

176 The following are statements regarding *Tinea nigra*:

T A. It is a superficial asymtomatic mycosis.
F B. It is more common in cold areas.
T C. Exophialia (Phaeoanellomyces) wernekii is an etiologic agent.
T D. Pigmented macules on palms or/ and soles are presentations.
T E. Direct microscopy of skin scrapings mounted in 10%

potassium hydroxide is diagnostic.

177   The following are statements regarding mycetoma:

T   A.   It is caused by a wide variety of free-living or exogenous aerobic actinomycetes.

T   B.   It is most prevalent in tropical and subtropical regions.

T   C.   Actinomycotic Mycetoma is presented as red grain.

T   D.   In Eumycotic Mycetoma the organisms appear as fungal hyphae 2-6 or more width.

F   E.   Actinomycotic Mycetoma is treated by Surgical excision or Amputation.

178   The following are statements regarding chromoblastomycosis:

T   A.   It is chronic, pruritic, progressive, indolent lesion.

T   B.   It is most common in tropical or subtropical areas especially in bare-footed agriculture workers.

T   C.   Cladophialophoracarrionii is causative agent.

F   D.   It is transmitted by person to person spread.

T   E.   Large papillomatous lesion involving large portion of the limb is a presentation.

179   The following are statements regarding sporotrichosis:

T   A.   It is chronic cutaneous or systemic mycosis caused by the thermally dimorphic fungus.

F   B.   It is transmitted by person to person.

T   C.   It is worldwide in distribution, but most in temperate as well as tropical region.

T   D.   Cutaneous form consisting of a linear chain of painless subcutaneous nodules.

T   E.   Systemic form is often localized in a single organ system.

180   The following are statements regarding infections by Aspergillus species:

F A. They occur in majority of patients who have prolonged neutropenia.

T B. *Aspergillus fumigatus* is the most frequently isolated species.

T C. They may occur locally at sites of intravenous catheter insertion.

T D. They produce painful skin nodules.

T E. Skin lesions resemble pyoderma gangrenosum lesions.

181 Risks for CNS infections include

T A. Extremes of age.
T B. Immunocompromised.
T C. Head Trauma.
F D. Labrotomy.
T E. Chronic alcoholi/cirrhosis.

182 The following CNS infections are correctly matched with their common causative agents:

T A. Bacterial meningitis : Pneumococcus.
T B. Viral meningitis   : Enteroviruses.
T C. Fungal meningitis   : Cryptococcus.
F D. Encephalitis   : Staph aureus.
T E. Brain abcess   : Anerobes.

183 The following are statements regarding viral menigitis:

F A. Age usually is above 40yo.
T B. Photophobia is a presentation.
T C. Enteroviruses are the main causative virus.
T D. Hematogenous spread to CNS is a route of infection.
T E. Normal glucose is a laboratory finding.

184 The following are statements regarding viral encephalitis:

T A. EBV is one of causative agents.
F B. Psychiatric presentations is clue for Herpes zoster etiology.

T   C.   Arboviruses are the common causative agent among parkinsonism patients.

F   D.   EEG is normal in viral encephalitis.

T   E.   MRI is used in diagnosis.

185   The following are statements regarding HSV encephalitis:

F   A.   Severe neurological defects occur in minority of patients.

T   B.   Nearly 1/3 of infections are primary infections.

T   C.   Affection of temporal lobes and frontal lobes produce the psychiatric features.

T   D.   Fever is a presentation in majority of patients.

F   E.   High protein is a laboratory finding of CSF.

186   The following are statements regarding viral meningitis:

T   A.   Herpes simplex virus is one of the causative agents.

T   B.   Enteroviruses are the most common causative viruses.

F   C.   More cases occur during the winter months.

T   D.   The inability to isolate bacterial pathogens in relation to viral meninigits has led to the term ''aseptic meningitis.

F   E.   The clinical course of most of types of viral meningitis is sever and lethal.

187   The following are statements regarding viral encephalitis:

T   A.   Rabies one of the causative agents.

F   B.   The arboviruses are transmitted through blood transfusions.

T   C.   Altered levels of consciousness is common clinical feature.

T   D.   Lumpur puncture often shows a picture compatible with aseptic meningitis.

T   E.   Only HSV disease has specific therapy available.

188   The following are statements regarding Prion disease in CNS:

T   A.   It aggregate extracellularly within the central nervous system to form plaques.

T   B.   The lesion is characterized by vacuole formation in the neurons.

F   C.   The incubation period for prion disease is relatively less than one month.

T   D.   The disease progresses rapidly, leading to brain damage and death.

T   E.   Astemizole has been found to have anti prion infection.

189   The following are statements regarding *Prion diseases in CNS*:

T   A.   They are transmissible spongiform encephalopathies.
T   B.   There are human and animal forms.
T   C.   They are rare.
T   D.   They cause neurodegeneration.
F   E.   They are self-limited diseases.

190   The following are statements regarding bacterial meningitis:

T   A.   Pneumococcus is the most common cause.
T   B.   Mortality 50 - 90% with severe initial neurologic impairment.
T   C.   Bacteria can cross BBB and enter CSF usually at choroid plexi/dural sinuses.
F   D.   Decreased CSF protein due to vascular permeability and leakage.
T   E.   Meningismus is a presentation in majority of cases.

191   Causal organism of aseptic meningitis include

F   A.   *Staphylococcus aureus.*
T   B.   *Leptospira interrogans.*
T   C.   *Polio virus.*
T   D.   *Treponema pallidum.*
F   E.   *Haemophillus influenza.*

192   The following are statements regarding investigations findings in bacterial meningitis:

T   A.   Increased wbc in CSF.

T   B.   Decrease glucose in CSF.

T   C.   Increased protein in CSF.

F   D.   If Gram stain -ve intracellular diplococci means the cause is Pneumococcus.

T   E.   If Gram stain -ve bacilli means the causative agent is Ecoli.

193   The following are statements regarding bacterial meningitis:

F   A.   Neisseria meningitides affect adults more than 45 years of age.

T   B.   The disease appears to occur in males more than females.

T   C.   The infectious organism first colonizes the nasopharynx..

T   D.   Rapid onset of fever is common clinical presentation.

T   E.   In most patients with bacterial meningitis, lumpur puncture can be safely performed without antecedent neuroimaging.

194   The following are statements regarding brain abscess:

F   A.   Brain abscess secondary to otitis media occur more frequently among young adults.

T   B.   Neck rigidity is rare.

T   C.   Ring-enhancing lesion with surrounding edema is the finding of CT scan.

F   D.   Lumpur puncture is help in diagnosis.

T   E.   Treatment is usually includes a third generation cephalosporin and metronidazole.

195   The following are statements regarding Tuberculous meningitis:

F   A.   Confusion is an early feature.

F   B.   Majority of patients with miliary TB have TB meningitis.

T   C.   Analysing of cerebrospinal fluid is diagnostic.

T   D.   The CSF usually has a high protein and low glucose.

T   E.   Hydrocephalus is a complication.

196   The following are statements regarding fungal meningitis:

T   A.   *Cryptococcus neoformans* is the cause.
T   B.   The infection is by inhalation.
F   C.   Rapid development of symptoms.
T   D.   Decreased glucose in CSF.
T   E.   Amphotericin B + 5-fluorocytosin is the drug of choice.

197   The following predisposing factors are correctly matched with the specific pathogen:

T   A.   Neonatal age   :   *E.coli.*
T   B.   Otitis media and sinusitis : *S.pneumoniae.*
T   C.   Penetrating head trauma or neurosurgery : *S.aureus.*
T   D.   Immunocompromised host : *Mycobacterium tuberculosis.*
T   E.   Endocarditis : *S.aureus.*

198   The following are statements regarding nosocomial infection:

T   A.   It is a clinical infection that was neither present nor was in its incubation period when the patient entered the hospital.
F   B.   Must make their appearance before discharge from the hospital.
T   C.   Low resistance of the patients is a risk factor..
F   D.   The source of the infecting organism should be only exogenous.
T   E.   Group A Streptococci is a common cause

199   The most common types of nosocomial infections are

T   A.   Surgical wound and other soft tissue infections.
T   B.   Urinary tract infections.
T   C.   Respiratory infections.
T   D.   Gastroenteritis.
F   E.   Encephalitis.

200   Factors most associated with an increased incidence of postoperative infections in the hospital are

T   A.   Over 60 years, of age.
T   B.   Preoperative stay in hospital.
T   C.   Long duration of the surgical procedure.
T   D.   Pre-existing infection at the site of the wound.
F   E.   Patient with uncontroled hypertension.

201   The following are statements regarding surgical wound infections:

T   A.   Treatment with depilatories has been associated with a much higher frequency of infection.
T   B.   Staphylococcus aureus is the dominant species.
T   C.   They occurs commonly at the time of surgery.
F   D.   The main origin of the bacteria is from a member of the surgical team.
T   E.   Aerial transmission is a coomon mode of spread of infections.

202   The causal agents of infective endocarditis include

T   A.   *Streptococcus mutans.*
T   B.   *Pseudomonas aeruginosa.*
T   C.   *Haemophilus* species.
T   D.   *Escherichia coli.*
F   E.   *Bordetella pertussis.*

203   The following are statements regarding infective endocarditis:

T   A.   The sets blood culture are positive.
T   B.   Staphylococci are causative organisms.
T   C.   Janeway lesions are located on the palms or soles of the patient.
F   D.   patient is afebrile.
F   E.   cystoscopy is a predisposing factor.

204   Factors affect the control of hospital infections

T   A.   The lack of quality control of sterilization and disinfection procedures.

T   B.   The quality of water and food made available in the hospital.

T   C.   The lack of trained staff.

T   D.   The lack of knowledge of hospital infection control principles and practices among the staff.

T   E.   The hospital environment itself.

205   The following nosocomial pathogens are correctly matched with its infection

T   A.   *Staphylococcus epidermidis* :   i.v. infections.

T   B.   *Escherichia coli*   :   urinary infections.

T   C.   MRSA *S. aureus*   :   Bone infections.

T   D.   *Pseudomonas* spp. :   GIT infection.

F   E.   *Legionella* species   :   diarrhoea.

206   The following are statements regarding roles of natural defense of the respiratory system:

T   A.   Epithelial layer of mucous memebrane secretes mucus which maintains moist surfaces and traps many microbes.

F   B.   Cilia on mucous membranes of upper respiratory tract move upwards towards throat.

T   C.   Nose hair filters dust, pollen, and microbes.

T   D.   Coughing and sneezing expel foreign objects.

T   E.   Lysozyme found in nasal secretions breaks down gram+ cell walls.

207   The following are statements regarding pathogens of the respiratory system:

T   A.   Respiratory pathogens are easily transmitted from human to human.

F   B.   All respiratory pathogens exist as part of the normal flora.

T   C.   *Legionella* only infects the lung.

T   D.   *Streptococcus* can cause infection in multiple sites of RT.

T   E.   Most dangerous fungi are *Aspergillus* and *Pneumocystis*.

208   The following bacteria is a common causative agent of following upper respiratory tract (URT)

T   A.   *Haemophilus influenzae* : Laryngitis.
T   B.   *Streptococcus pneumoniae* : Epiglottitis.
T   C.   *Streptococcus pyogenes.* : Otitis media.
F   D.   *Streptococcus pyogenes* : sinusitis.
T   E.   *Streptococcus pyogenes* : Pharyngitis.

209   The following are statements regarding pharyngitis:

F   A.   Bacterial pharyngitis is more common than viral.
T   B.   Epstein–Barr virus is a causative of viral pharyngitis.
T   C.   Red pharyngeal mucosa is a presentation.
T   D.   Peak incidence of bacterial type is during the rainy season in the tropics.
F   E.   Viral pharyngitis is treated by antiviral drug.

210   The following are statements regarding common cold:

T   A.   It is a frequent occurrence, especially in young children.
F   B.   Its peak incidence during the winter period.
F   C.   The condition is caused mainly by *Streptococcus pyogenes*.
T   D.   Nasal discharge is a presentation.
F   E.   It is treated by antibiotics.

211   Pneumocystis pneumonia

T   A.   is caused by *Pneumocystis jirovecii.*
F   B.   causes life-threatening pneumonia amongimmunocompetent person.
T   C.   is common in patients with AIDS when the CD4 cell counts drop below 200/mm^3.
T   D.   causal agent has charateristics of both protozoan and fungus.
F   E.   treated with tetracycline.

212   The following are statements regarding influenza:

T A. It is caused by influenza virus groups A–C.
T B. Myalgia is common presentation.
F C. Diagnosis is usually by laboratory investigation.
T D. *Staphylococcus aureus* can cause secondary bacterial pneumonia.
F E. A vaccine is available, but it is only effective against newly isolated strains.

213 The following are statements regarding otitis media:

F A. It is an inflammation of external auditory meatus.
T B. Infection is most often caused by *S. pneumoniae* or *H. influenzae*.
T C. It is most frequent in the younger child, whose Eustachian tube is shorter and more horizontal.
T D Fever is a common feature.
F E. Meningitis is a common complication. .

214 The following are statements regarding acute sinusitis:

T A. It is most commonly caused by *S. pneumoniae* and *H. influenzae*.
T B. There is impaired drainage of sinus secretions as a result of a prior upper respiratory tract infection or similar cause.
T C. Headache is a presentation.
F D Diagnosis is mainly by organism isolation.
F E. Treatment is mainly by oral antibiotics.

215 The following are statements regarding laryngitis:

T A. It is caused by one of the 'respiratory' viruses.
T B. There is swelling and irritation of the voice box.
T C. It is associated with hoarseness and loss of voice.
T D. It may also be a feature of a common cold or influenza.
F E. Specific antiviral therapy is required.

216   The following are statements regarding bronchitis:

T   A.   Acute bronchitis is caused by *M. pneumonia*.
T   B.   *H. influenzae* is cause of cute exacerbation of chronic bronchitis.
T   C.   *S.pneumoniae* is a causative agent of Tracheobronchitis.
F   D.   Sputum culture is of high diagnostic value.
T   E.   Oral ampicillin is used in treatment.

217   The following are statements regarding scarlet fever:

F   A.   It is caused by *Streptococcus pyogenes*.

T   B.   It is usually seen in children under age of 18 years.
T   C.   Symptoms usually begin with appearance of a rash.
T   D.   Lymphadenopathy in neck is a finding.
T   E.   It is treated by antibiotic therapies.

218   The following are statements regarding :

T   A.   It is caused by the toxin produced by *Corynebacterium diphtheria*.
T   B.   Can be accompanied by plaque-like pseudomembrane in the throat.
T   C.   It is transmitted by direct contact with skin.
T   D.   Effects of infection are due to the exotoxin.
F   E.   It is difficult to treat it by antibiotics.

219   The following are statements regarding viral infections of the upper respiratory tract:

T   A.   There are four types of single-stranded enveloped RNA parainfluenza virus.
T   B.   Transmission and pathology of parainfluenza virus similar to influenza virus.
F   C.   Parainfluenza is a serious problem in adults.
T   D.   Rhinoviruses are extremely small, non-enveloped, single-stranded RNA viruses.

T   E.   Picornavirus infect nasopharynx because it has the same temperature for growth (33°C).

220 Bacterial infections of the lower respiratory tract include

T A. Chlamydial pneumonia.
T B. *Legionella* pneumonia.
T C. Pertussis.
T D. Inhalation anthrax.
F E. Scarlet fever.

221 The following are statements regarding bacterial pneumonia:

T A. It is characterized by inflammation of the alveoli and abnormal alveolar filling with fluid.
T B. Cough is a typical symptom.
T C. *Klebsiella pneumoniae* is one of causative agents.
T D. Establishment of an infection in the lungs depends on the number of pathogens entering and the competence of the mucociliary escalator.
T E. Bacterial pneumonia is treated with antibiotics.

222 The following pneumonias caused by different bacteria are correctly matched with clinical features:

T A. *Streptococcus pneumoniae* : Sudden onset pleuritic pain, fever, rusty sputum, cold sores.
T B. *Klebsiella pneumoniae* : Thick, viscous red sputum, alcoholic patient.
T C. *Staphylococcus aureus* : Pneumonia following influenza.
T D. *Streptococcus pneumoniae :* Pneumonia in the chronic bronchitic.
F E. *Mycoplasma pneumoniae* : Upper lobe consolidation, hilar lymphadenopathy, vagrant or alcoholic.

223 The following are statements regarding mycoplasma pneumonia:

T	A.	It is caused by *Mycoplasma pneumonia.*
F	B.	It is severe form of pneumonia.
T	C.	Accounts for about 10% of all pneumonias.
F	D.	Most common age for infections is between 20 and 40 years.
T	E.	Erythromycin is the drug of choice.

224 The following are statements regarding hospital-acquired pneumonia:

T	A.	It is the third most common nosocomial infection.
F	B.	Legionellas is the most common cause.
T	C.	Purulent sputum is a presentation.
T	D.	Bronchoalveolar lavage is the preferred method for collection of bacteriological specimens.
F	E.	Many patients respond well to optimal antimicrobial therapy.

225 Common bacterial causes of nosocomial pneumonia include

T	A.	*Staphylococcus aureus.*
F	B.	*Streptococcus pneumoniae.*
T	C.	*Pseudomonas aeruginosa.*
F	D.	*Mycobacterium tuberculosis.*
T	E.	*Klebsiella pneumonia.*

226 The following are statements regarding pulmonary tuberculosis:

T	A.	Chronic pneumonia is a common presentation of *M. tuberculosis.*
T	B.	It is common throughout the developing world.
T	C.	Primary infection follows airborne transmission from an individual with pulmonary tuberculosis.
F	D.	The thin cell wall of mycobacteria renders the organisms resistant to phagocytosis.
T	E.	Primary tuberculous pneumonia only occurs if cell-mediated immunity is inadequate to resist the initial infective challenge.

OSMAN, AYE, WISMAN, GHADA

227 The following are statements regarding diagnosis of pulmonary tuberculosis:

T   A.   Clinically fever, night sweats, weight loss and haemoptysis are all should be clinical features.

T   B.   The radiographic appearance supports one of the clinical presentations.

T   C.   Routine Gram stain should be used.

T   D.   Ziehl–Neelsen stain is acid fast stain .

F   E.   The culture identification and susceptibility results take 48 hours.

228 The following are statements regarding pathogenesis of tuberculosis:

T   A.   *M. tuberculosis* cell wall interferes with macrophage function.

T   B.   *M. tuberculosis* cell wall inhibits the formation of the phagolysosome.

T   C.   *M. tuberculosis* escape into the cytoplasm where it increases in number & eventually spreads to the lymph nodes.

T   D.   Primary tuberculosis follows initial exposure to the pathogen.

F   E.   Secondary tuberculosis occurs few weeks after the primary TB.

229 The following are statements regarding primary tuberculosis:

T   A.   It occurs when a host encounters pathogen for the first time.

T   B.   Organisms find their way to the alveoli when a localized inflammatory response develops.

F   C.   Pathogens are coomonly killed in the alveoli.

F   D.   The type of immune response is mainly humoral immune response.

T   E.   Tubercles are aggregates of enlarged macrophages filled with bacteria.

230 The following are statements regarding secondary

tuberculosis:

T   A.   It can be due to reactivation of old lesions.

T   B.   It could be due to gradual progression of primary tuberculosis into chronic disease.

F   C.   The incidence occur in majority of patients.

T   D.   It usually manifests itself in the apices of the lung.

T   E.   It usually occurs within two years of the primary infection.

231   The following are statements regarding pertussis:

T   A.   It is caused by *Bordetella pertussis.*

T   B.   The causative bacteria does not survive in the environment.

T   C.   Symptoms can be similar to those of a cold.

F   D.   Mortality is lowest in infants and children under 1 year old.

T   E.   Greatest numbers of infections are among 10-20 year-olds.

232   The following are statements regarding empyema:

T   A.   It is the accumulation of purulent fluid in the pleural space.

T   B.   Infection resulting from penetrating thoracic trauma is a route.

T   C.   Enterobacteriaceae is one of the causative agents.

F   D.   The collection of pus is required for diagnosis.

T   E.   It is treated by heavy antibotics.

233   The following are statements regarding inhalation anthrax:

F   A.   The causative agent *Bacillus anthracis.*is a gram-negative rod.

T   B.   It produces a fulminate pneumonia comes on suddenly with great severity.

T   C.   Antiphagocytic properties of the capsule aid its survival and growth in large numbers.

T   D.   It leads to respiratory failure.

T   E.   It is used recently as a biological weapon.

234   The following are statements regarding viral infections of the lower respiratory tract:

T   A.   They cause majority of all acute respiratory tract infections.
F   B.   Greatest incidence is among adults.
T   C.   Influenza virus is a cause of majority of them.
T   D.   Short incubation period of 1 to 4 days is a common characteristics of infection.
T   E.   Direct transmission is through droplets.

235   The following are statements regarding fungal infections of the respiratory system:

T   A.   *Pneumocystis (carinii) jiroveci is a cause of a lethal pneumonia common in AIDS patients.*
F   B.   *Pneumocystis (carinii) jiroveci* is easily grown in culture.
F   C.   Blastomycosis is increased in AIDS.
T   D.   Fever, chills, and drenching sweats are presentation of blastomycosis.
T   E.   Histoplasmosis affects people who live and work in the vicinity of bat or bird droppings.

236   The following are statements regarding aspergillosis:

T   A.   Invasive aspergillosis shows a rapid progression to death.
T   B.   Typically seen in the immunocompromised patients.
T   C.   Fungus produces extracellular proteases, phospholipases, and toxic metabolites.
T   D.   Seen more in nosocomial infections associated with air-conditioning systems.
F   E.   Hemoptysis is absent in this infection.

237   The following are statements regarding infections of gastrointestinal tract:

T   A.   Exogenous infections are brought in with contaminated food or water.

T   B.   *C. difficile* and other exogenous infections are frequently acquired in hospital environments.

T   C.   Exogenous infections can cause nausea and vomiting within 6 hours.

T   D.   Endogenous infections are caused by organisms that are part of the normal flora.

F   E.   *Streptococcus* is an example of exogenous infections.

238   The following are statements regarding *Enterobacteriaceae*:

T   A.   O antigen is lipopolysaccharide in the outer membrane.

T   B.   K antigen is surface polysaccharides.

T   C.   H antigens are falgella proteins of motile strains.

F   D.   Most of them colonize the upper gastrointestinal tract.

F   E.   *Shigella* and *Salmonella* are part of the normal flora.

239   The following are statements regarding enteric fever:

T   A.   It is a systemic infection focused in the gastrointestinal tract.

T   B.   Abdominal pain is a prominent feature.

F   C.   Diarrhea is severe from the 1st day of the infection.

T   D.   Pathogenesis involves the penetration of enterocytes.

T   E.   Pathogens spread to organs of the reticuloendothelial system.

240   The following are statements regarding typhoid fever:

T   A.   It is caused by *Salmonella enterica* serotype Typhi.

T   B.   The chronic carriers are the primary reservoir.

F   C.   *S. Typhi* survive for short period inside viable host macrophages.

T   D.   Systemic infection is exacerbated by release of lipopolysaccharide endotoxin.

T   E.   The entire cycle takes only two weeks.

241   The following are statements regarding typhoid fever:

T   A.   It is caused by invasive infection from small intestine into blood stream.

T B. *Salmonella typhi* multiply in phagocytes resulting in septicemia.

F C. Bacteria produce only exotoxin.

T D. Transmitted by contaminated water or food.

T E. Treated by broad spectrum antibiotic.

242 Toxin type of food poisoning can be caused by

F A. *Salmonella Typhi.*

T B. *Bacillus cereus.*

T C. *Clostridium perfringens.*

T D. *Staphylococcus aureus.*

F E. *Streptococcus pyogenes.*

243 The following are statements regarding enteric fever:

F A. E. The stool culture is useful for the diagnosis during first week of illness.

F B. F. It is caused by *Salmonella Typhi* only.

T C. G. It can present with pea soup diarrhea.

T D. H. It is transmitted by the house flies.

T E. Intestinal perforation is one of the complications.

244 The following are statements regarding typhoid fever:

F A. The temperature rises rapidly in the first week.

T B. Diarrhea can occur in the second week of onfection.

T C. Intestinal perforation in the distal ileum is a complication.

T D. It spread through poor hygiene habits.

T E. Widal test is a diagnostic.

245 The following are statements regarding salmonella gastroenteritis:

F A. It occurs in the intestine.

T B. It results from improper food handling.

T C. The chronic carriers are an important reservoir.

T   D.   *Salmonella enterica* can withstand the phagocytic response.

T   E.   Transcytosis and the inflammatory response cause the onset of diarrhea.

246   The following are statements regarding cholera:

F   A.   Cholera is an infection of the large intestine caused by the bacterium *Vibrio cholera.*

T   B.   Watery diarrhea is a main symptoms.

T   C.   Transmission occurs primarily by drinking water or eating contaminated food of an infected person.

T   D.   A rapid dip-stick test is to determine the presence of *V. cholera.*

T   E.   Oral rehydration therapy is the primary treatment.

247   The following are statements regarding cholera:

T   A.   It is caused by Gram negative curved rod.

T   B.   *V. cholerae* can grow in fresh or salt water.

F   C.   *V. cholerae* causes disease by release of exotoxin.

T   D.   Vaccine is inadequate to prevent the disease.

F   E.   Antibiotic therapy is the primary treatment.

248   The following are statements regarding Vibrio:

T   A.   It is highly motile by means of a single polar flagella.

T   B.   It can grow either aerobically or anaerobically.

F   C.   It has high tolerance for acidic conditions Grow well in mildly alkaline environments.

T   D.   Cell structure similar to that of Gram-negative bacteria.

T   E.   Its toxin causes a devastating intestinal infection.

249   The following are statements regarding Escherichia coli infection:

T   A.   Caused by Gram negative coliform.

T   B.   *Escherichia coli* commonly found as normal flora,

T   C.   Types of infection vary depending on the presence and type of exotoxins.

F D Shiga-like toxins can result in mild diarrhea and nausea.
.

T E. Treatment by rehydration and controversial antibiotic treatment.

250 The following are statements regarding bacterial infections of GIT:

T A. *Streptococcus mutans* is one of the causes.
T B. *Helicobacter pylori* cause gastritis.
T C. *Clostridium difficile* causes antibiotic-associated enterocolitis.
T D. Toxins *of Clostridium difficile* produce pseudomembranes made up of fibrin and cells.
F E. Toxins produced by S.aureus causes slowly progressive gastroenteritis.

251 Most common bacterial foodborne pathogens are

T A. *Campylobacter jejuni.*
T B. *Clostridium perfringens.*
T C. *Salmonella* spp.
T D. *Escherichia coli.*
F E. *Brucella* spp.

252 The following are statements regarding food poisoning:

T A. It appear suddenly and within 48 hours after ingestion of food contaminated with a pathogen.
T B. Abdominal cramping is symptom.
T C. Infective agents include viruses, bacteria, and parasites.
F D. Food poisoning caused by Salmonella bacteria gives victims flu-like symptoms for as long as 48 hours.
F E. Staphylococcal food poisoning appears about 48 hours after eating contaminated food.

253 Symptoms of food poisoning include:

T   A.   Abdominal cramps.
T   B.   Diarrhea (may be bloody).
T   C.   Fever and chills.
F   D.   Severe abdominal pain.
T   E.   Nausea and vomiting.

254   The following are statements regarding food poisoning:

T   A.   *Staphylococcus aureus* enterotoxin is a superantigen.
F   B.   Diarrhea caused by *Staphylococcus aureus* is a typical feature of this kind of food poisoning.
T   C.   *B. cereus* is associated with reheated fried rice.
T   D.   Ingestion of *B. cereus* exotoxin produces mild symptoms.
T   E.   Shiga toxin causes inflammation and bleeding.

255   The following are statements regarding food poisoning:

T   A.   Infectious agents include viruses, bacteria, and parasites.
T   B.   Toxic agents include fungal toxins (poisonous mushrooms).
F   C.   Low -level contamination with salmonella may result in a food poisoning-like syndrome.
T   D.   Mortality of Salmonella spp due to septic shock caused by endotoxin.
T   E.   *Campylobacter jejuni* usually transmitted in cow's milk and related products.

256   The following are statements regarding *Helicobacter pylori*:

T   A.   They are similar to *Campylobacter* in morphology and growth characteristics.
F   B.   Lipopolysaccharides in the outer layer is less toxic than those in other Gram-negative pathogens.
T   C.   Production of a urease Allows it to survive in very acidic environments.
T   D.   It produces a vacuolating cytotoxin.
T   E.   Infected cells have large vacuoles throughout their cytoplasm.

257   The following are statements regarding peptic ulcer caused by
Helicobacter pylori:

T   A.   *Helicobacter pylori* has multiple polar knobbed flagella.
T   B.   Urease is a virulence factor of bacteria.
F   C.   Weight gain is a presentation.
T   D   Diagnosed by assessing damage to stomach lining and
    .   isolation of urease+, Gram- vibrios.
T   E.   Perforations of stomach or intestine is a complication.

258   The following are statements regarding watery diarrhea:

T   A.   It is caused by enterotoxin-secreting bacteria.
T   B.   Enterotoxigenic *Escherichia coli is cause.*
F   C.   Watery diarrhea caused by *V. cholerae* uasually resolve in 3
         to 7 days.
T   D.   May be accompanying by vomiting and fever.
T   E.   Usually self-limiting.

259   The following are statements regarding traveler's diarrhea:

T   A.   Enterotoxigenic strains of *E. coli.* Is acause.
F   B.   Majority are caused by *Shigella..*
T   C.   Usually brief and self-limiting.
T   D.   The major source is ingestion of improperly cooked food.
T   E.   Typically involves multiple patients.

260   The following are statements regarding nosocomial
gastrointestinal infections:

T   A.   E. coli is one of a major causative pathogen.
T   B.   Contaminated food prepared outside the hospital is a source.
T   C.   *C. difficile* accounts for 90% of infections.
F   D.   Symptoms are usually only mild diarrhea.
T   E.   Colitis arises either during or after treatment with
         antibiotics.

261   The following are statements regarding shigella:

F   A.   Shigella is like E.coli both can ferment lactose.
T   B.   *S. dysenteriae* produces most of Shiga toxin.
T   C.   Shigellosis is one of the most common causes of diarrhea worldwide.
T   D.   *S. dysenteriae* causes bacillary dysentery.

T   E.   There is direct connection between *Shigella* infections and community sanitary practices.

262   The following are statements regarding pathogenesis of shigellosis:

F   A.   *Shigella* is affected by human gastric acid.
T   B.   *Shigella* causes mucosal ulcerations and abscess formation.
T   C.   There is cell-to-cell extensions cause localized ulcers in the mucosa, particularly in colon.
T   D.   *Shigella* lyses the vacuole membranes.
F   E.   Shiga toxin causes less severity of the illness.

263   The following are statements regarding Campylobacter enteritis:

T   A.   It is caused by *Campylobacter jejuni*.
F   B.   The primary reservoir is human.
T   C.   Undercooked poultry is the most common source.
T   D.   Bacteria adhere to and enter cells in endocytic vacuoles.
F   E.   Illness begins about 2 weeks after ingestion includes fever and lower abdominal pain.

264   The following are statements regarding viral infections of the digestive system:

T   A.   Diarrhea is the most common sign of infection.
F   B.   Diarrhea lasts for at least 30 days.
T   C.   There is abundant excretion of virions in the stool.
T   D.   Virus must be detected in ill patients.

T   E.   Must be has a significant antibody response.

265 Specific criteria must be met to implicate viruses in digestive infections include:

F   A.   Virus must be detected in non-ill and ill patients.
T   B.   Viral shedding must correlate with onset of symptoms.
T   C.   Disease must be reproduced by experimental inoculation of non-immune humans or animals.
T   D.   Must be a significant antibody response.
T   E.   Other causes of the signs and symptoms must be excluded.

266 Viruses that can cause gastrointestinal infections are

T   A.   Rotavirus.
T   B.   Calicivirus.
T   C.   Astrovirus.
T   D.   Some serotypes of adenovirus.
T   E.   Enterovirus.

267 The following are statements regarding Rotavirus:

F   A.   It is enveloped spherical virus.
T   B.   It has a double-capsid structure.
F   C.   It is a cause of less than 10% of cases of acute gastroenteritis.
F   D.   Outbreaks of rotavirus infections common in adults.
T   E.   Malabsorption is the end result of infection.

268 The following are statements regarding Enterovirus:

T   A.   Enteroviruses are members of the *picornaviridae*.
T   B.   They can survive in the stomach.
T   C.   Humans are the natural hosts.
F   D.   Symptomatic infection is common.
T   E.   Virus will normally spend 1 to 4 weeks in the oropharynx.

269   The following are statements regarding Hepatitis A:

T   A.   It is classified as a member of the genus *hepatovirus*, family *picornaviridae.*

F   B.   It is non-enveloped, double-stranded RNA virus.

F   C.   They have many serotype.

T   D.   Transmission is usually via the fecal-oral route.

T   E.   Seen in feces 10-14 days before onset of symptom.

270   The following are statements regarding Hepatitis A:

T   A.   Virus replicates initially in intestinal mucosa.

T   B.   It causes necrosis of the parenchymal cells.

F   C.   Patients with antibodies can be reinfected.

T   D.   Incubation times vary from 10 to 50 days,

T   E.   Stool can become clay-colored 1 to 5 days before onset of jaundice.

271   The following are statements regarding Hepatitis B:

F   A.   It is classified as a member of family *picornaviridae.*

T   B.   It is a DNA virus.

T   C.   It has spherical shape with a surrounding envelope.

T   D.   Its envelope contains viral surface antigens HBsAg.

T   E.   It is used as a template for reverse transcription.

272   The following are statements regarding Hepatitis B infection:

F   A.   Majority of those infected become chronic carriers.

T   B.   50% of infections are sexually transmitted.

T   C.   Tattooing or piercing can easily transmit this viral infection.

T   D.   Lesions in acute hepatitis B infections resemble those seen with other hepatitis viruses.

T   E.   Screening of blood donors has markedly reduced the incidence of transfusion transmission.

273   The following are statements regarding Hepatitis B infection:

T   A.   Incubation time is 7-160 days.
T   B.   Loss of appetite is a presentation of acute infection.
T   C.   Chronic active infection causes a continued inflammation resulting in necrosis of hepatocytes.
T   D.   Progressive fibrosis is a finding.
F   E.   Majority of infected individuals will develop chronic hepatitis.

274   The following are statements regarding Hepatitis C:

T   A.   Classified as a member of the *flaviviridae* family.
F   B.   It is DNA virus.
T   C.   It has six major genotypes and multiple subtypes.
T   D.   It transmitted by blood transfusions.
T   E.   Hemodialysis patients are also at risk.

275   The following are statements regarding Hepatitis C:

F   A.   Incubation time is 4-6 weeks.
F   B.   Infection is usually severe.
T   C.   Majority of those infected will become carriers of the infection.
T   D.   Hepato cellular carcinoma is a late consequences of chronic hepatitis C infection.
T   E.   Hepatitis C is the leading cause of liver transplants.

276   The following are statements regarding Hepatitis D:

F   A.   It is double-stranded DNA virus.
F   B.   It requires the presence of hepatitis C.
T   C.   Seen most often in intravenous drug abusers.
T   D.   Recurrence of jaundice occurs in superinfection with hepatitis D.
T   E.   Interferon-α is given to doubly infected patients.

277   The following are statements regarding Hepatitis E:

T   A.   It is classified in the family *caliciviridae.*
F   B.   It is non-enveloped DNA virus.
T   C.   It is transmitted by the fecal-oral route.
T   D.   Infection is frequently subclinical.
T   E.   The incubation time is about 40 days.

278   The following are statements regarding Hepatitis G:

T   A.   Classified in the family *flaviviridae.*
F   B.   It is similar to hepatitis B.
T   C.   RNA virus.
T   D.   2% of blood donors are positive for hepatitis G RNA.
T   E.   No treatment is available.

279   The infection which associated with the strain of *Escherichia coli* include:

T   A.   Neonatal meningitis.
T   B.   Urinary tract infection.
T   C.   Haemolytic uraemic syndrome.
F   D   Bacillary dysentery.
.
F   E.   Enteric Fever.

280   The following bacteria that biochemically ferment with lactose sugar include

T   A.   *Esherichia coli.*
F   B.   *Salmonella typhi.*
F   C.   *Shigella boydii.*
T   D.   *Klebsiella pneumonia.*
F   E.   *Pseudomonas aeruginosa.*

281   Following infections can be transmitted from mother to fetus via placenta.

F	A.	Typhoid.
F	B.	Malaria.
T	C.	Syphilis.
T	D.	AIDS.
T	E.	Rubella.

282   Common uropathogens include

T	A.	*Escherichia coli.*
T	B.	*Proteus.*
T	C.	*Pseudomonas aeruginosa.*
F	D.	*Mycobacterium tuberculosis.*
T	E.	*Staphylococcus aureus.*

283   Commensal microflora of the urethra include

F	A.	*Staphylococci saprophyticus.*
T	B.	*Viridans and non-hemolytic streptococci.*
T	C.	*Lactobacilli.*
F	D.	*Corynebacterium urealyticum.*
T	E.	*Saprophytic Neisseria.*

284   Common risk factors for urinary tract infection in women

T	A.	Urinary tract obstruction.
F	B.	Hypertension.
T	C.	Pregnancy.
T	D.	Sexual intercourse.
T	E.	Estrogen deficiency.

285   Common risk factors for urinary tract infection in men include

T	A.	Urinary tract obstruction.
T	B.	Prostatic enlargement.
T	C.	Urologic instrumentation or surgery.
F	D.	Hydrocele.
T	E.	Lack of circumcision.

286   The following are statements regarding UTI:

F   A.   Hematogenous route of infection is the most common.
T   B.   Colonization of urethra and periurethral tissue by uropathogens the initial event.
T   C.   Hospital infection associated with lower urinary tract instrumentation.
T   D.   Enteric bacteria is source of uropathogens.
T   E.   Papillary necrosis: complication of pyelonephritis.

287   The following are statements regarding bacterial virulence factors in UTI:

T   A.   *Escherichia coli* strains expressing O-antigens cause high proportion of infections.
T   B.   Gram-negative endotoxin decreases ureteral peristalsis.
F   C.   K6 antigens of *E. coli* associated with antiphagocytic activity.
T   D   P-fimbriated *E. coli* is a cause of pyelonephritis.
.
T   E.   *Hemolysin* produced by many uropathogens damages renal tubular epithelium and promotes invasive infection.

288   The following are statements regarding host protective factors in UTI:

T   A.   Flushing mechanism of micturition.
T   B.   Low vaginal pH (3.5-4.5) suppresses colonization by uropathogens.
T   C.   Normal acid pH of urine (4.6-6) is anti-bacterial
F   D   Urinary Tamm-Horsefall protein blocks *Staph aureas*
.   attachment to uroepithelial cells..
T   E.   Chemotactic interleukin-8 eradicate bacteriuria

289   The following are statements regarding signs and symptoms of UTI:

F   A.   Fever is high in lower UTI.

T B. Frequent and painful urination in lower UTI.
T C. Occasional suprapubic pain or sensation of heaviness in lower UTI.
T D. Flank pain is present in upper UTI.
T E. Fever and chills in upper UTI.

290 Indications for urinalysis and culture

T A. Symptoms suggestive of infection like dysuria.
T B. Suspicion of complicated infection as fever.
T C. Atypical symptoms.
T D. Failure to respond to initial therapy.
F E. Recurrent symptoms < 2 weeks after treatment for a previous UTI not cultured.

291 Factors affecting growth & colony count of bacteria in urine

T A. Urine pH.
T B. Urine constituents.
T C. Urine flow rate.
T D. Residual urine volume.
T E. Urinary antiseptics.

292 Anaerobic infections

T A. can be associated with gas in tissues.
T B. are usually present with foul-smelling discharge.
F C. are rarely associated with contamination of normal flora.
T D. are sometimes polymicrobial nature.
F E. cannot be treated with antimicrobial drugs.

293 The following microorganism can cause urinary tract infection.

T A. *Candida albicans.*
F B. *Streptococcocus agalactiae.*
F C. *Salmonella Typhi.*
T D. *Escherichia coli.*

T   E.   *Staphylococcus saprophyticus.*

294   The following are statements regarding non-gonoccocal urethritis (NGU) :

T   A.   Chlamydia trachomatis accounts for a majority of NGU.
F   B.   One of the implicated organism in NGU is *Haemophilus influenzae.*
F   C.   *Rickettsia prowazekii* infection leads to severe form of NGU.
T   D.   Serology (ELISA/Latex agglutination test) is the mainstay for diagnosing NGU.
T   E.   The majority of NGU cases are asymptomatic.

295   Microorganisms which can be used as potential biological weapon include

T   A.   *Brucella abortus.*
F   B.   *Leptospira interrogans.*
T   C.   *Yersinia pestis.*
T   D.   *Bacillus anthracis.*
F   E.   *Mycobacteria leprae.*

296   The following are statements regarding diagnostic tests of UTI:

T   A.   Bacterial count >100,000 /ml indicative of infection in urinanalysis.
F   B.   Nitrite dipstick test the presence of protein.
T   C.   Leukocyte esterase test identifies WBC in urine.
T   D.   Gram stain of urine is obtained by clean catch urine.
T   E.   Urine culture and sensitivity identify infecting organism and most effective antibiotic.

297   The following are statements regarding diagnostic tests for adults who have recurrent infections or persistent bacteriuria:

T   A.   Intravenous pyelography (IVP) evaluates structure and excretory function of kidneys, ureters, and bladder.

F B. Barium enema is used to visualize the internal structures.

T C. Voiding cystourethrography is to assess bladder and urethra when filled and during voiding.

T D. Cystoscopy is used for diagnostic, tissue biopsy, interventions.

T E. Manual pelvic or prostate examinations to assess structural changes of genitourinary tract.

298 The following are statements regarding possible outcomes of treatment for UTI, determined by follow-up urinalysis and culture:

T A. Cure; no pathogens in urine.

T B. Unresolved bacteriuria.

T C. Persistent bacteriuria or relapse.

T D. Development of new infection with different pathogen.

F E. No pathogen bacteria with a lot of WBS.

299 The following are statements regarding urethritis:

T A. It is often associated with sexually transmitted pathogens.

T B. Frequency is presentation.

F C. Painless urination is a presentation.

T D. Urine is cloudy.

T E. Treatment start when microorganism counts is 100,000/ml.

300 The following are statements regarding acute cystitis:

T A. It is caused mainly by E. coli.

F B. Painless urination is a presentation.

F C. The incidence among men more than women.

T D. Urine is cloudy and malodorous.

T E. Leukocyte esterase positive.

301   The following are statements regarding acute pyelonephritis:

T   A.   Blood stream is a route of invasion.
T   B.   Both kidneys are always affected.
F   C.   Fever and chills are common presentations.
T   D   Leukocytosis is present.
        .
T   E.   It require IV antibiotics.

302   The following are statements regarding chronic pyelonephritis:

T   A.   It is a chronic tubulointerstitial inflammation involving renal parenchyma.
T   B.   Leads to scarring of pelvis and calyces.
T   C.   Chronic inflammatory infiltrates.
F   D   Decrease incidence of preterm labor in pregnancy.
        .
T   E.   Papillary necrosis is a complication.

303   The following are statements regarding catheter-associated UTI:

T   A.   Long term catheter bacteriuria is inevitable.
T   B.   40% of nosocomial infections.
F   C.   Most common source of gram-positive bacteremia.
T   D   Asymptomatic bacteriuria should not treated unless they are
        .   immunosuppressed.
T   E.   Severe infection needs IV antibiotics.

304   The following are statements regarding pregnancy and urinary tract infections:

T   A.   There is increased risk of kidney infections in pregnancy.
F   B.   During pregnancy, high progesterone levels elevate the risk of symptomatic bacteriuria.
F   C.   If bacteriuria is present they do have a high risk of a kidney infection.
T   D   A kidney infection during pregnancy may result in premature

.   birth or pre-eclampsia.

T   E.   Treatment is recommended when urine testing shows signs of an infection even in the absence of symptoms.

305   The following are statements regarding fungal urinary tract infections:

T   A.   Candida albicans is the most common cause.
T   B.   Diabetes is a predisposing factors
F   C.   Ascending infection is common
T   D   Urine urine leukocytosis is a finding.

T   E.   Urine fungal culture catheterization for fungal culture is used in diagnosis.

306   Nosocomial pathogens include

T   A.   *Clostridium difficile.*
T   B.   *Staphylococcus aureus.*
F   C.   *Clostridium tetani.*
F   D   *Helicobacter pylori.*

T   E.   *Pseudomonas aeruginosa.*

307   The following are statements regarding vaginitis and vaginosis:

T   A.   Symptoms depend on the etiologic agent.
T   B.   *Candida albicans* is initially normal biota living in low numbers.
T   C.   White vaginal discharge occurs in *Candida albicans* infection.
T   D   Vaginal discharge with a very fishy odor, especially after sex is characteristic of ifection by *Gardnerella* species.
F   E.   Itching is uncommon in *Gardnerella* species.

308   The following are statements regarding gonorrhea:

T   A.   *N. gonorrhoeae* is the etiologic agent.

F   B.   It is commonly spread from the urethra to epididymis in male patients.

F   C.   It leads to infertility in majority of infected men.

T   D.   Mucopurulent or bloody vaginal discharge is a presentation in women.

T   E.   Pelvic inflammatory disease is a compication in women.

309   The following are statements regarding gonorrhea:

T   A.   It is caused by bacteria *Neisseria gonorrhea.*

F   B.   It is leading cause of sterility in men.

T   C.   Endocarditis is a complication.

T   D.   It is diagnosed by a smear of the discharge.

T   E.   It is treated with antibiotics.

310   The following are statements regarding gonorrhea:

T   A.   Majority of women asymptomatic carriers.

T   B.   May cause Pelvic Inflammatory Disease (PID) in women.

T   C.   Man develops a drip, pus exudate 3-8 days after exposure

F   D.   Painful urination in women

T   E.   If newborn has contact with the bacteria during birth may cause blindness

311   Specific serological tests for syphilis are

F   A.   VDRL test

T   B.   FTA-ABS test.

T   C.   EIA.

T   D.   TPI test.

F   E.   Rapid plasma reagin test.

312   The following are statements regarding Chlamydia:

F   A.   Majority of cases are symptomatic.

T   B.   Symptoms mimicking gonorrhea in male patients.
T   C.   Cervicitis is a presentation in women.
F   D.   All strains can invade the lymphatic tissues resulting in lymphogranuloma venereum.
T   E.   Babies born to mothers with infections can develop eye infections and pneumonia.

313   The following are statements regarding classification of sexually-transmitted diseases:

T   A.   *Gonorrhea* is a mucosal infection.
F   B.   Papillomavirus is a systemic infections.
T   C.   HIV is a systemic infections.
T   D.   Herpes simplex is ulcerative infections.

T   E.   Chancroid is ulcerative infections.

314   Factors that affect the transmission of STDs

T   A.   Age.
T   B.   Gender.
T   C.   Genetic susceptibility.
F   D.   Smoking.

T   E.   Circumcision in males.

315   The following are statements regarding chlamydial infection:

F   A.   It affects young adults more than teenagers.
T   B.   It may have been acquired in the remote past.
F   C.   Around 5% of infected sexual partners in males.
T   D.   ~ 50% of infected sexual partners in women.

T   E.   Urethritis occurs in both males and females.

316   The following are statements regarding microbiology of gonorrhea:

T   A.   It is strict human pathogen.
F   B.   It is Gram-positive diplococcus
T   C.   IgA protease (cleaves IgA).
T   D.   Oxidase-positive.

T   E.   Fastidious growth.

317   Virulence determinants of Neisseria gonorrhoeae include:

T   A.   Pilus colonization factor.
T   B.   Opa proteins.
T   C.   Lipooligosaccharide.
T   D.   IgA1 protease.

T   E.   Transferrin.

318   The following are statements regarding *Chlamydia trachomatis*:

T   A.   It is obligate intracellular bacteria.
F   B.   It is Gram negative bacteria.
T   C.   It has 2-stage life cycle.
T   D.   Reticulated body is vegetative like.

T   E.   Treated by tetracycline.

319   The following are statements regarding syphilis causative bacteria:

T   A.   *Treponema pallidum* is a spirochete and labile spiral bacterium.
F   B.   Man and animal are recognized hosts.
T   C.   It is non-cultivable bacteria.
T   D.   It is Gram-negative like.

T   E.   It has axial filaments.

320   The following are statements regarding microbiology of chancroid:

T   A.   It is caused by *Haemophilus ducreyi*.
F   B.   Gram-positive coccobacilli.
T   C.   Fastidious and labile.
T   D.   Diagnosis is usually clinical, by exclusion of other agents of genital ulcers.
F   E.   Females >> Males.

321   The following are statements regarding pelvic inflammatory disease:

F   A.   It is caused by gonorrhea only.
T   B.   It is an infection of the fallopian tubes, uterus and ovaries.
T   C.   It causes sterility in women.
T   D.   There is scarring of fallopian tubes lead to ectopic pregnancies.
T   E.   Treated with antibiotics.

322   The following are statements regarding genital warts:

T   A.   HPV types 6 and 11 are most frequently the cause of genital warts.
F   B.   It increased the risk for endometrial cancer.
T   C.   Warts on genitalia 2 weeks to 8 months after exposure.
T   D.   It is spread through direct skin-to-skin contact.
F   E.   Genital warts are commonly occur singly.

323   The following are statements regarding Herpes genitalis:

T   A.   Refers to a genital infection by Herpes simplex virus.
T   B.   Most individuals carrying herpes are unaware about the infection.
F   C.   Genital HSV-2 infections are the cause of majority of infections.
T   D.   Herpes is asymptomatic in the majority of cases.
T   E.   In males, the lesions occur on the glans penis.

324   The following are statements regarding genital Herpes in women:

T   A.   Increase chance of miscarriages.

T   B.   Increase cervical cancer risk.

F   C.   The treatment eradicates the symptome and viruses.

T   D.   Stress leads to reoccurs at times.

T   E.   Acyclovir is the drug of choice.

325   The following are statements regarding human papillomavirus (HPV):

F   A.   It is an RNA virus from the papillomavirus family.

F   B.   Majority of the known types of HPV cause symptoms in most people.

T   C.   Most HPV infections in young women are temporary and have little long-term significance.

T   D.   There is high risk of developing precancerous lesions of the cervix.

T   E.   High-risk sexually transmitted HPVs lead to the development of cervical intraepithelial neoplasia (CIN).

5 MEDICAL PARASITOLOGY

5.1 Questions without answers: (True/False questions):

326   The following are general concepts in parasitology:

   A.   By definition, all vectors are arthropods.
   B.   All trematodes require at least one snail intermediate host.
   C.   Some cestodes have separate sexes.
   D.   Protozoa are simple organisms with one nucleus.
   E.   A criterion used in the classification of protozoa is the structure used for movement.

327   The following are statements regarding parasites::

   A.   Parasites may require more than one host to complete its life cycle.
   B.   Protozoa without locomotive structures are classified as

Sporozoa.
C.   Helminths in Greek means worms.
D.   Flukes are bilaterally symmetrical.
E.   Flukes are not found in the lungs.

328   The following are statements regarding parasites:

A.   'Metazoa' refers to organisms with changing shapes.
B.   Most trematodes look like leaves.
C.   All cestodes have both sexes in one organism.
D.   Sporozoa are ciliated spores.
E.   Flagellates may be found in the lymphatics.

329   Examples of parasitic mechanisms of disease include

A.   production of allergenic substances by *Ascaris lumbricoides.*
B.   obstruction of the large gut by *Trichuris trichiura.*
C.   interference with fat absorption by *Hymenolepis nana.*
D.   formation of pipestem fibrosis by *Schistosoma japonicum.*
E.   formation of space-occupying lesions by *Echinococcus granulosus.*

330   Mosquitoes are the vector in the following disorders

A.   onchocerciasis.
B.   visceral leishmaniasis.
C.   Loasis.
D.   African trypanosomiasis .
E.   Malayan filariasis.

331   Scabies

A.   is caused by a 6-legged arthropod.
B.   is more common amongst pet owners.
C.   of the Norwegian type occurs most commonly in immunocompromised people.
D.   lesions are typically found on the face and palms of the hand.
E.   is usually diagnosed clinically.

332   Cutaneous larva migrans

A.   is also known as creeping eruption.
B.   is caused by animal tapeworms.
C.   is characterized by itchy and painful serpiginous tracks of the skin.
D.   is usually diagnosed by detecting high eosinophilia.
E.   can be treated with thiabendazole.

333   The following are statements regarding vivax malaria:

A.   The causative parasite invades mainly old red blood cells.
B.   The clinical manifestations are usually more severe than those of falciparum malaria.
C.   It causes quotidian fever.
D.   The ameboid trophozoite is the typical diagnostic stage of the parasite.
E.   Primaquine is effective against hypnozoites.

334   The following are statements regarding falciparum malaria:

A.   The causative parasite invades mainly young red blood cells.

B.   It is more severe in pregnant women.

C.   The presence of schizonts in the peripheral blood indicates severe infection.

D.   Its recurrence after the acute attack is caused by hypnozoites in the liver.

E.   It is the only type of malaria to cause complications.

335   The following are statements regarding the pathogenesis and clinical manifestations of malaria:

A.   The pre-erythrocytic liver cycle may cause jaundice.

B.   Hypersplenism may be caused by autoimmunity.

C.   The presence of schizonts of Plasmodium falciparum in peripheral blood   indicates poor prognosis.

D.   In cerebral malaria, hypoxia is caused by capillary sludging due to red cell stickiness.

E.   Plasmodium malariae infection does not cause any complications.

336   The following are statements regarding the treatment of malaria:

A.   Schizontocides relieve the febrile paroxyms.

B.   To prevent transmission, the trophozoites need to be eradicated from the blood.

C.   Quinghaosu may be used in the presence of chloroquine resistance.

D.   Quinine is contraindicated in Orang Asli with G6PD

deficiency.

E.   Pregnant women should not be given treatment until after delivery.

337   Lymphatic filariasis

A.   is primarily found in Asia and the tropics.

B.   is transmitted to humans through mosquito bites.

C.   presents as periodic fever in the early stage.

D.   is characterized by the presence of microfilaria in the blood during the stage of elephantiasis.

E.   is treated with diethylcarbamazine (DEC).

338   The following are recognised features of onchocerciasis:

A.   keratitis.

B.   diarrhoea.

C.   "hanging groin".

D.   Calabar swelling.

E.   eosinophilia.

339   Loa loa

A.   is confined to Central and West Africa.

B.   is spread by the mosquitoes.

C.   may cause blindness.

D.   is diagnosed by histological examination of skin snips.

E.   is treated with DEC.

340   The following are statements regarding African

trypanosomiasis:

A.   It has an incubation period of 4-6 months.
B.   It may cause erythema chronicum migrans in light skinned persons.
C.   The Gambian form progresses more rapidly.
D.   The Gambian form is associated with a more prominent chancre.
E.   The Gambian form can be treated with pentamidine.

341   The following occur in Chagas' disease (American trypanosomiasis):

A.   Lymphadenopathy.
B.   Meningoencephalitis.
C.   Calabar swelling.
D.   Mega-oesophagus.
E.   Saddle-nose deformity.

342   Visceral leishmaniasis is typically caused by

A.   *Leishmania donovani.*
B.   *Leishmania.tropica.*
C.   *Leishmania chagasi.*
D.   *Leishmania major.*
E.   *Leishmania infantum.*

343   Giardiasis

A.   is transmitted via contaminated food and drink.
B.   leaves the small bowel morphologically normal.

C. is associated with rice-water stool.

D. can be diagnosed by duodenal biopsy.

E. usually responds to treatment with metronidazole.

344 The following are statements regarding ascariasis:

A. Most infections are asymptomatic.

B. Migration of the adult worms to the lungs causes Loeffler's syndrome.

C. A single worm may cause complications.

D. Worm bolus may be clinically confused with appendicitis.

E. Light infection may be detected by culture technique.

345 Hookworm

A. is usually spread by the faeco-oral route.

B. may block the pancreatic duct causing pancreatitis.

C. eggs can be readily distinguished microscopically from those of *Strongyloides* sp.

D. causes hypochromic microcytic anaemia in charonic cases.

E. infection is treated with albendazole.

346 Strongyloidiasis

A. may occurs in temperate regions.

B. may present with diarrhea with blood and mucus.

C. may cause hyperinfection in immunocompromised patients.

D. is diagnosed by detecting eggs in feces.

E. may be treated with thiabendazole.

347   Trichuriasis

A.   may be a problem in urban communities.
B.   is one of the causes of Loeffler's syndrome.
C.   is associated with pruritus around the perianal area.
D.   is confirmed by the detection of worm eggs which look like rugby balls.
E.   is better treated with pyrantel pamoate than albendazole.

348   The following are statements regarding enterobiasis:

A.   It is caused by the threadworm.
B.   Inhalation is one of the modes of infection.
C.   It causes serious pathology in the colon.
D.   Pruritus ani is a common manifestation.
E.   Proper sanitation is a preventive strategy.

349   *Entamoeba histolytica*

A.   trophozoites contain ingested red blood cells.
B.   produces cysts in the lower part of the colon.
C.   forms sinuses in the colon.
D.   infection is usually confined to the colon.
E.   may be treated with thiabendazole.

350   Amoebic liver abscess:

A.   mainly occurs in developing countries.
B.   usually affects the right lobe of the liver.
C.   is associated with eosinophilia.

D.   should be aspirated routinely.

E.   should be treated by diloxanide furoate alone.

351   Flatworms infecting the liver include

A.   *Clonorchis sinensis.*

B.   *Paragonimus westermani.*

C.   *Fasciolopsis buski.*

D.   *Schistosoma japonicum.*

E.   *Echinococcus granulosus.*

352   The following are statements regarding *Schistosoma haematobium* infection:

A.   The bladder mucosa is unaffected.

B.   Hematuria is a common presentation.

C.   Hydronephrosis is seen In chronic infection.

D.   Bladder carcinoma is frequently seen as a late complication.

E.   Inflammatory fibrotic reactions to retained eggs cause chronic disease.

353   Trichomoniasis

A.   is a sexually transmitted disease.

B.   presents with vaginal discharge associated with pruritus.

C.   is diagnosed by presence of trophozoites in the vaginal discharge.

D.   should be suspected in a patient with non-gonococcal urethritis.

E.   is treated with nystatin cream.

354   **The following are statements regarding toxoplasmosis:**

A.   Congenital infection is more serious than the acquired infection.

B.   Choroidoretinitis is an early presentation in infected neonates.

C.   The presence of IgG antibody confirms the infection in neonates.

D.   Encephalitis is particularly common in adult AIDS patients.

E.   Sulfadiazine and pyrimethamine are used in combination to treat adults.

355   **The following are pairs of parasites and the diseases they cause in the nervous system:**

A.   *Acanthamoeba* spp: amebic keratitis.

B.   *Naegleria* spp: primary amebic meningo-encephalitis.

C.   *Trypanosoma cruzi*: sleeping sickness.

D.   *Echinococcus granulosus*: hydatidosis.

E.   *Necator americanus*: hyperinfection syndrome.

356   **The following source of infection are correctly paired:**

A.   Freshwater fishes: *Clornorchis sinensis* .

B.   Freshwater plants: *Fasciola hepatica* .

C.   Contaminated soil: *Enterobius vermicularis* .

D.   Undercooked beef: *Fasciolopsis buski* .

E.   Crab and crayfishes: *Paragonimus westermani* .

357   Parasites that need two intermediate hosts are

A.   *Paragonimus westermani* .
B.   *Taenia* spp.
C.   *Schistosoma* spp.
D.   *Clornorchis sinensis.*
E.   *Echinococcus granulosus* .

358   Arthropods

A.   literally mean "jointed legs".
B.   are defined as " invertebrates with bodies that are divided into head, thorax and abdomen.
C.   which develop via hemimetabolous life cycles have stages which look different from each other.
D.   can be used in forensic investigations.
E.   are not very successful from the evolutionary standpoint.

359   The following are statements regarding protozoa:

A.   The nuclei of amoebae aid in the identification of species.
B.   All tissue protozoa are transmitted by vectors.
C.   Some intestinal flagellates are transmitted in the form of trophozoites.
D.   The pathology caused by the intestinal ciliate is limited to the intestinal lumen.
E.   Blastocystis hominis is classified under the protozoa.

360   Fever, diarrhea and eosinophilia in a returned traveler may be due to infections caused by

A.   *Strongyloides stercoralis.*
B.   *Aeromonas hydrophilia* .
C.   *Schistosoma mansoni* .
D.   *Capillaria philippinensis.*
E.   *Plasmodium falciparum* .

361   The following pairs are true of the parasitic infections and their treatment

A.   Onchocerciasis: ivermectin .
B.   Schistosomiasis: praziquantel.
C.   Leishmaniasis: suramin.
D.   Trypanosomiasis: pentavalent antimony.
E.   Hydatid disease: albendazole.

362   Praziquantel is used in the treatment of

A.   Amoebiasis.
B.   Toxocariasis (visceral larva migrans) .
C.   Paragonimiasis .
D.   Trypanosomiasis .
E.   Schistosomiasis.

363   The following are statements regarding parasites and their location in the hosts during infestations:

A.   *Ascaris lumbricoides*:   small intestines .
B.   *Clonorchis sinensis*: bile ducts .
C.   *Taenia solium*:lungs .
D.   *Dracunculus medinensis*: subcutaneous tissue .

E.   *Schistosoma haematobium*:meninges .

364   The following are statements regarding parasites and their modes of transmission:

A.   Schistosoma japonicum: Cercaria penetrate the skin in snail-infested water.
B.   Strongyloides stercoralis: Larvae penetrate through the skin.
C.   Taenia saginata: Ingestion of uncooked beef.
D.   Trichinella spiralis: Ingestion of eggs from fecal-contaminated food.
E.   Trichuris trichiura : Ingestion of uncooked pork.

365   Parasites cause harm to their hosts through

A.   obstruction.
B.   malabsorption .
C.   lymph loss.
D.   tissue damage .
E.   granuloma.

366   The following are statements regarding helminths:

A.   Helminths are either round or flat on cross-section.
B.   Cestodes are characterized by their body segments.
C.   The filarial worm is an example of a blood fluke.
D.   All trematodes have both sexes in one organism.
E.   Nematodes can be transmitted via contact with the soil.

367   The following are statements regarding trematodes (flukes):

A.   Their life cycle usually does not require an intermediate hosts.

B.   Paragonimus westermani infects the lungs.

C.   All are hermaphroditic except Schistosoma.

D.   Infections can be acquired by ingesting encysted cercariae in fish.

E.   Infections can be treated with Praziquantel.

368   The following are statements regarding mechanical vector:

A.   It carries the parasite on the surface of its body.

B.   It is essential in the life cycle of a parasite.

C.   It serves as a temporary "vehicle of transport".

D.   Its role in the transmission of disease is incidental.

E.   The prate undergoes sexual reproduction within it.

369   The following are statements regarding host-parasite relationships:

A.   An obligatory parasite can live outside its host.

B.   A transport host can support the development of parasites.

C.   'Symbiosis' means 'living together'.

D.   Only humans can be dead-end hosts.

E.   A vector is an arthropod host which transmits disease.

370   Parasites cause disease in the following manner:

A.   Malaria parasites attack white blood cells.

B.   The common round worms may block the intestine.

C.   A ciliate can cause sexually-transmitted disease.

D.   Free-living amebas attack the brain.

E.   Maggots burrow tunnels in the skin.

371   The following are correct pairs of poisonous arthropods and their venom apparatus:

A.   Scorpions: pedipalps.

B.   Bees: ovipositor.

C.   Caterpillars: body hairs .

D.   Centipedes: chelicerae.

E.   Spiders: pincers.

372   The following are statements regarding pediculosis:

A.   It occasionally occurs in temperate countries.

B.   For transmission to occur, there must be direct skin contact.

C.   Pthiriasis is considered as a sexually-transmitted disease.

D.   Heavy infestation may cause anemia.

E.   Gamma benzene hexachloride is the treatment of choice for children.

373   The following are statements regarding scabies:

A.   Transmission occurs as a result of contact with animals.

B.   The infective stage is the female mite.

C.   The lesions are mostly localized to specific parts of the body.

D.   The diagnosis is usually based on its clinical manifestations.

E.   Benzyl Benzoate in the usual dose is suitable for babies.

374   The following are statements regarding myiasis:

A.   It is diagnosed by detecting maggots in ulcers.
B.   The posterior spiracle of the maggot is used for species identification.
C.   Infested wound has to be bandaged until the maggots die.
D.   It is also known as larva migrans.
E.   Albendazole is the drug of choice.

375   The following principles apply in the diagnosis of parasitic infections:

A.   Occasionally, clinical diagnosis is adequate to begin treatment.
B.   The timing of specimen collection is sometimes important.
C.   In real-life practice, all specimens need to be stained before the laboratory   can make a diagnosis.
D.   The main laboratory strategy is to identify the causative agents.
E.   Immunological techniques are more reliable than simple staining methods.

5.1 Questions with answers: (True/False questions) :

326   The following are general concepts in parasitology:

T   A   By definition, all vectors are arthropods.
    .

T   B.   All trematodes require at least one snail intermediate host.

F   C.   Some cestodes have separate sexes.

F   D   Protozoa are simple organisms with one nucleus.
    .

T   E.   A criterion used in the classification of protozoa is the structure used for movement.

327   The following are statements regarding parasites::

T   A   Parasites may require more than one host to complete its life
    .   cycle.

T   B.   Protozoa without locomotive structures are classified as Sporozoa.

T   C.   Helminths in Greek means worms.

T   D   Flukes are bilaterally symmetrical.
    .

F   E.   Flukes are not found in the lungs.

328   The following are statements regarding parasites:

F   A   'Metazoa' refers to organisms with changing shapes.
    .

T   B.   Most trematodes look like leaves.

T   C.   All cestodes have both sexes in one organism.

F   D   Sporozoa are ciliated spores.
        .

F   E.   Flagellates may be found in the lymphatics.

329   Examples of parasitic mechanisms of disease include

T   A.   production of allergenic substances by *Ascaris lumbricoides*.

F   B.   obstruction of the large gut by *Trichuris trichiura*.

F   C.   interference with fat absorption by *Hymenolepis nana*.

T   D.   formation of pipestem fibrosis by *Schistosoma japonicum*.

T   E.   formation of space-occupying lesions by *Echinococcus granulosus*.

330   Mosquitoes are the vector in the following disorders

F   A.   onchocerciasis.

F   B.   visceral leishmaniasis.

F   C.   Loasis.

F   D.   African trypanosomiasis .

T   E.   Malayan filariasis.

331   Scabies

F   A.   is caused by a 6-legged arthropod.

F   B.   is more common amongst pet owners.

T   C.   of the Norwegian type occurs most commonly in immunocompromised people.

F   D.   lesions are typically found on the face and palms of the hand.

T   E.   is usually diagnosed clinically.

332   Cutaneous larva migrans

T   A.   is also known as creeping eruption.
F   B.   is caused by animal tapeworms.
T   C.   is characterized by itchy and painful serpiginous tracks of the skin.
F   D.   is usually diagnosed by detecting high eosinophilia.
T   E.   can be treated with thiabendazole.

333   The following are statements regarding vivax malaria:

F   A.   The causative parasite invades mainly old red blood cells.
F   B.   The clinical manifestations are usually more severe than those of falciparum malaria.
F   C.   It causes quotidian fever.
F   D.   The ameboid trophozoite is the typical diagnostic stage of the parasite.
F   E.   Primaquine is effective against hypnozoites.

334   The following are statements regarding falciparum malaria:

F   A.   The causative parasite invades mainly young red blood cells.
T   B.   It is more severe in pregnant women.
T   C.   The presence of schizonts in the peripheral blood indicates severe infection.
F   D.   Its recurrence after the acute attack is caused by hypnozoites in the liver.
F   E.   It is the only type of malaria to cause complications.

335 The following are statements regarding the pathogenesis and clinical manifestations of malaria:

F A. The pre-erythrocytic liver cycle may cause jaundice.

T B. Hypersplenism may be caused by autoimmunity.

T C. The presence of schizonts of Plasmodium falciparum in peripheral blood indicates poor prognosis.

T D. In cerebral malaria, hypoxia is caused by capillary sludging due to red cell stickiness.

F E. Plasmodium malariae infection does not cause any complications.

336 The following are statements regarding the treatment of malaria:

T A. Schizontocides relieve the febrile paroxyms.

F B. To prevent transmission, the trophozoites need to be eradicated from the blood.

T C. Quinghaosu may be used in the presence of chloroquine resistance.

T D. Quinine is contraindicated in Orang Asli with G6PD deficiency.

F E. Pregnant women should not be given treatment until after delivery.

337 Lymphatic filariasis

T A. is primarily found in Asia and the tropics.

T B. is transmitted to humans through mosquito bites.

F   C.   presents as periodic fever in the early stage.

F   D.   is characterized by the presence of microfilaria in the blood during the stage of elephantiasis.

T   E.   is treated with diethylcarbamazine (DEC).

338   The following are recognised features of onchocerciasis:

T   A.   keratitis.

F   B.   diarrhoea.

T   C.   "hanging groin".

F   D.   Calabar swelling.

T   E.   eosinophilia.

339   Loa loa

T   A.   is confined to Central and West Africa. (T)

F   B.   is spread by the mosquitoes.

F   C.   may cause blindness.

F   D.   is diagnosed by histological examination of skin snips.

T   E.   is treated with DEC.

340   The following are statements regarding African trypanosomiasis:

F   A.   It has an incubation period of 4-6 months.

F   B.   It may cause erythema chronicum migrans in light skinned persons.

F   C.   The Gambian form progresses more rapidly.

F   D.   The Gambian form is associated with a more prominent chancre.

T   E.   The Gambian form can be treated with pentamidine.

341 **The following occur in Chagas' disease (American trypanosomiasis):**

T A. Lymphadenopathy.
T B. Meningoencephalitis.
F C. Calabar swelling.
T D. Mega-oesophagus.
F E. Saddle-nose deformity.

342 **Visceral leishmaniasis is typically caused by**

T A. *Leishmania donovani.*
F B. *Leishmania.tropica.*
T C. *Leishmania chagasi.*
F D. *Leishmania major.*
T E. *Leishmania infantum.*

343 **Giardiasis**

T A. is transmitted via contaminated food and drink.
F B. leaves the small bowel morphologically normal.
F C. is associated with rice-water stool.
T D. can be diagnosed by duodenal biopsy.
T E. usually responds to treatment with metronidazole.

344 **The following are statements regarding ascariasis:**

T A. Most infections are asymptomatic.
F B. Migration of the adult worms to the lungs causes

Loeffler's syndrome.

T   C.   A single worm may cause complications.

T   D.   Worm bolus may be clinically confused with appendicitis.

F   E.   Light infection may be detected by culture technique.

345   Hookworm

F   A.   is usually spread by the faeco-oral route.

F   B.   may block the pancreatic duct causing pancreatitis.

F   C.   eggs can be readily distinguished microscopically from those of *Strongyloides* sp.

T   D.   causes hypochromic microcytic anaemia in charonic cases.

T   E.   infection is treated with albendazole.

346   Strongyloidiasis

T   A.   may occurs in temperate regions.

T   B.   may present with diarrhea with blood and mucus.

T   C.   may cause hyperinfection in immunocompromised patients.

F   D.   is diagnosed by detecting eggs in feces.

T   E.   may be treated with thiabendazole.

347   Trichuriasis

T   A.   may be a problem in urban communities.

F   B.   is one of the causes of Loeffler's syndrome.

F   C.   is associated with pruritus around the perianal area.

T   D.   is confirmed by the detection of worm eggs which look like rugby balls.

F   E.   is better treated with pyrantel pamoate than albendazole.

348   The following are statements regarding enterobiasis:

F   A.   It is caused by the threadworm.

T   B.   Inhalation is one of the modes of infection.

F   C.   It causes serious pathology in the colon.

T   D.   Pruritus ani is a common manifestation.

F   E.   Proper sanitation is a preventive strategy.

349   *Entamoeba histolytica*

T   A.   trophozoites contain ingested red blood cells.

T   B.   produces cysts in the lower part of the colon.

F   C.   forms sinuses in the colon.

F   D.   infection is usually confined to the colon.

F   E.   may be treated with thiabendazole.

350   Amoebic liver abscess:

T   A.   mainly occurs in developing countries.

T   B.   usually affects the right lobe of the liver.

F   C.   is associated with eosinophilia.

F   D.   should be aspirated routinely.

F   E.   should be treated by diloxanide furoate alone.

351   Flatworms infecting the liver include

T   A.   *Clonorchis sinensis.*

F   B.   *Paragonimus westermani.*

F   C.   *Fasciolopsis buski.*

T   D.   *Schistosoma japonicum.*

T   E.   *Echinococcus granulosus.*

352   The following are statements regarding *Schistosoma haematobium* infection:

F   A.   The bladder mucosa is unaffected.
T   B.   Hematuria is a common presentation.
T   C.   Hydronephrosis is seen In chronic infection.
T   D.   Bladder carcinoma is frequently seen as a late complication.
T   E.   Inflammatory fibrotic reactions to retained eggs cause chronic disease.

353   Trichomoniasis

T   A.   is a sexually transmitted disease.
T   B.   presents with vaginal discharge associated with pruritus.
T   C.   is diagnosed by presence of trophozoites in the vaginal discharge.
T   D.   should be suspected in a patient with non-gonococcal urethritis.
T   E.   is treated with nystatin cream.

354   The following are statements regarding toxoplasmosis:

T   A.   Congenital infection is more serious than the acquired infection.
F   B.   Choroidoretinitis is an early presentation in infected neonates.
F   C.   The presence of IgG antibody confirms the infection in neonates.

T   D.   Encephalitis is particularly common in adult AIDS patients.

T   E.   Sulfadiazine and pyrimethamine are used in combination to treat adults.

355   **The following are pairs of parasites and the diseases they cause in the nervous system:**

T   A.   *Acanthamoeba* spp: amebic keratitis.

T   B.   *Naegleria* spp: primary amebic meningo-encephalitis.

F   C.   *Trypanosoma cruzi*: sleeping sickness.

T   D.   *Echinococcus granulosus*: hydatidosis.

F   E.   *Necator americanus*: hyperinfection syndrome.

356   **The following source of infection are correctly paired:**

T   A.   Freshwater fishes: *Clornorchis sinensis* .

T   B.   Freshwater plants: *Fasciola hepatica* .

F   C.   Contaminated soil: *Enterobius vermicularis* .

F   D.   Undercooked beef: *Fasciolopsis buski* .

T   E.   Crab and crayfishes: *Paragonimus westermani* .

357   **Parasites that need two intermediate hosts are**

T   A.   *Paragonimus westermani* .

F   B.   *Taenia* spp.

F   C.   *Schistosoma* spp.

T   D.   *Clornorchis sinensis.*

F   E.   *Echinococcus granulosus* .

358   Arthropods

T   A.   literally mean "jointed legs".

F   B.   are defined as " invertebrates with bodies that are divided into head, thorax and abdomen.

F   C.   which develop via hemimetabolous life cycles have stages which look different from each other.

T   D.   can be used in forensic investigations.

F   E.   are not very successful from the evolutionary standpoint.

359   The following are statements regarding protozoa:

T   A.   The nuclei of amoebae aid in the identification of species.

F   B.   All tissue protozoa are transmitted by vectors.

T   C.   Some intestinal flagellates are transmitted in the form of trophozoites.

F   D.   The pathology caused by the intestinal ciliate is limited to the intestinal lumen.

T   E.   Blastocystis hominis is classified under the protozoa.

360   Fever, diarrhea and eosinophilia in a returned traveler may be due to infections caused by

T   A.   *Strongyloides stercoralis.*

F   B.   *Aeromonas hydrophilia .*

T   C.   *Schistosoma mansoni .*

T   D.   *Capillaria philippinensis.*

F   E.   *Plasmodium falciparum .*

361   The following pairs are true of the parasitic infections and their treatment

T   A.   Onchocerciasis: ivermectin .

T   B.   Schistosomiasis: praziquantel.

F   C.   Leishmaniasis: suramin.

F   D.   Trypanosomiasis: pentavalent antimony.

T   E.   Hydatid disease: albendazole.

362   Praziquantel is used in the treatment of

F   A.   Amoebiasis.

F   B.   Toxocariasis (visceral larva migrans) .

T   C.   Paragonimiasis .

F   D.   Trypanosomiasis .

T   E.   Schistosomiasis.

363   The following are statements regarding parasites and their location in the hosts during infestations:

T   A.   *Ascaris lumbricoides*:   small intestines .

T   B.   *Clonorchis sinensis*: bile ducts .

F   C.   *Taenia solium*:lungs .

T   D.   *Dracunculus medinensis*: subcutaneous tissue .

F   E.   *Schistosoma haematobium*:meninges .

364   The following are statements regarding parasites and their modes of transmission:

T   A.   Schistosoma japonicum: Cercaria penetrate the skin in snail-infested water.

T   B.   Strongyloides stercoralis: Larvae penetrate through the skin.

T   C.   Taenia saginata: Ingestion of uncooked beef.

F   D.   Trichinella spiralis: Ingestion of eggs from fecal-contaminated food.

F   E.   Trichuris trichiura : Ingestion of uncooked pork.

365   **Parasites cause harm to their hosts through**

T   A.   Obstruction.

T   B.   Malabsorption .

F   C.   Lymph loss.

T   D.   Tissue damage .

T   E.   Granuloma.

366   **The following are statements regarding helminths:**

T   A.   Helminths are either round or flat on cross-section.

T   B.   Cestodes are characterized by their body segments.

F   C.   The filarial worm is an example of a blood fluke.

F   D.   All trematodes have both sexes in one organism.

T   E.   Nematodes can be transmitted via contact with the soil.

367   **The following are statements regarding trematodes (flukes):**

F   A.   Their life cycle usually does not require an intermediate hosts.

T   B.   Paragonimus westermani infects the lungs.

T   C.   All are hermaphroditic except Schistosoma.

T   D.   Infections can be acquired by ingesting encysted cercariae in fish.

T   E.   Infections can be treated with Praziquantel.

368   **The following are statements regarding mechanical vector:**

T   A.   It carries the parasite on the surface of its body.

F   B.   It is essential in the life cycle of a parasite.

T   C.   It serves as a temporary "vehicle of transport".

T   D.   Its role in the transmission of disease is incidental.

F   E.   The prate undergoes sexual reproduction within it.

369   **The following are statements regarding host-parasite relationships:**

F   A.   An obligatory parasite can live outside its host.

F   B.   A transport host can support the development of parasites.

T   C.   'Symbiosis' means 'living together'.

T   D.   Only humans can be dead-end hosts.

T   E.   A vector is an arthropod host which transmits disease.

370   **Parasites cause disease in the following manner:**

F   A.   Malaria parasites attack white blood cells.

T   B.   The common round worms may block the intestine.

F   C.   A ciliate can cause sexually-transmitted disease.

T   D.   Free-living amebas attack the brain.

F   E.   Maggots burrow tunnels in the skin.

371   **The following are correct pairs of poisonous arthropods and their venom apparatus:**

F   A.   Scorpions: pedipalps.

T   B.   Bees: ovipositor.

T C. Caterpillars: body hairs .
F D. Centipedes: chelicerae.
F E. Spiders: pincers.

372 The following are statements regarding pediculosis:

T A. It occasionally occurs in temperate countries.
F B. For transmission to occur, there must be direct skin contact.
T C. Pthiriasis is considered as a sexually-transmitted disease.
T D. Heavy infestation may cause anemia.
F E. Gamma benzene hexachloride is the treatment of choice for children.

373 The following are statements regarding scabies:

F A. Transmission occurs as a result of contact with animals.
T B. The infective stage is the female mite.
F C. The lesions are mostly localized to specific parts of the body.
T D. The diagnosis is usually based on its clinical manifestations.
F E. Benzyl Benzoate in the usual dose is suitable for babies.

374 The following are statements regarding myiasis:

T A. It is diagnosed by detecting maggots in ulcers.
T B. The posterior spiracle of the maggot is used for species identification.
F C. Infested wound has to be bandaged until the maggots die.
F D. It is also known as larva migrans.
F E. Albendazole is the drug of choice.

375   The following principles apply in the diagnosis of parasitic infections:

T   A.   Occasionally, clinical diagnosis is adequate to begin treatment.

T   B.   The timing of specimen collection is sometimes important.

F   C.   In real-life practice, all specimens need to be stained before the laboratory   can make a diagnosis.

T   D.   The main laboratory strategy is to identify the causative agents.

F   E.   Immunological techniques are more reliable than simple staining methods.

ABOUT THE AUTHORS

Dr. Muhamed T. Osman; PhD, presently, is Associate Professor of Pathology and Head of Pathology Department in Faculty of Medicine and Defence Health, National Defence University of Malaysia (UPNM). He was Consultant Pathologist and Clinical Lecturer at Teaching Laboratories, Medical City of Baghdad, Iraq and Senior Lecturer of Pathology at Universiti Teknologi MARA (UiTM) Malaysia. He is the author of eight books and has published more than 70 papers in peer reviewed journals.

Dr. Aye Aye Mon; MSc, presently, is Associate Professor of Medical Microbiology in Faculty of Medicine and Defence Health, UPNM Malaysia. She is member and associate fellow of Australasian College of Tropical Medicine, Queensland, Australia. She was the Head of Microbiology department in University of Medical Technology, Myanmar and Senior Lecturer, in University of Malaya, and SEGi University, Malaysia. She is engaging with publication of books, journal articles, research and teaching.

Dr. Mohammad Wisman Abdul Hamid; MSc, presently is Medical Lecturer and Head of Parasitology Unit in Faculty of Medicine and Defence Health, UPNM Malaysia. He received his M.D from University Science of Malaysia (USM) and earned his Master of Medical Science in Parasitology and Medical Entomology from National University of Malaysia (UKM).

Dr. Ghada I. Al-Duboni; PhD, presently is Assistant Professor of Medical Microbiology and Immunology, in the Department of Basic Sciences, College of Dentistry, University of Baghdad, Iraq. She is engaging with publication of journal articles, research and teaching.